HEALTHCARE

STRATEGIC

PLANNING

Approaches for

the 21st Century

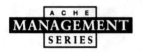

Alan M. Zuckerman

HEALTHCARE

STRATEGIC

PLANNING

Approaches for

the 21st Century

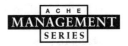
ACHE
MANAGEMENT
SERIES

Health Administration Press   Chicago, Illinois

02   01   00   99   98   5   4   3   2

Library of Congress Cataloging-in-Publication Data

Zuckerman, Alan M.
    Healthcare strategic planning: approaches for the 21st century
/ Alan M. Zuckerman.
        p.   cm.
Includes bibliographical references.
ISBN 1-56793-068-9
        1. Health facilities—Administration.   2. Strategic planning.
    I. Title.
RA971.Z79   1998   97-29506
362.1'068—dc21   CIP

The paper used in this publication meets the minimum require-ments of American National Standard for Information Sciences—Permanence of Paper for Printed Library Materials, ANSI Z39.48-1984. ∞™

Health Administration Press
A division of the Foundation
    of the American College of
    Healthcare Executives
One North Franklin
Suite 1700
Chicago, IL 60606
312/424-2800

iv

Contents

Acknowledgments

LIKE MOST people, I never imagined that I would write a book. When Health Administration Press called last year to ask me to write a text on healthcare strategic planning, I was both flattered and fearful. Despite having written dozens of articles and with lots of material and 25 years of experience in healthcare strategic planning, could I really write a book and did I have enough to say that would be worthwhile to others? On the latter point, you will certainly be the judge of that.

While I remain solely responsible for the content of this text, many people played important roles in bringing this project to fruition.

At the outset, Ted Druhot and my prolific aunt and uncle, Midge and Norman Podhoretz, encouraged me to get started and provided tips on how to work through writer's block.

My contributing authors, Justin Doheny, Karl Bartscht, Susan Sargent, and my silent contributor, Jack Campbell, helped assemble the case studies that are an important part of the book.

At the back end, my colleague, Jim Lifton, helped reshape some quite disparate material into coherent chapters.

Throughout this book, Susan Arnold, my editorial assistant, has been of invaluable help in ways too numerous to mention. It is impossible to imagine how this book would have been completed without Susan's active participation and support.

I received support from my former consulting firm, Chi Systems, throughout the manuscript development process. The office staff in Chi Systems' Philadelphia office labored silently, diligently, and purposefully through my reams of handwritten text and oddly configured charts, tables, and other figures. Christine Passaglia, in particular, deserves special thanks for doing the lion's share of interpretation of my scribbles and transforming them into readable text.

Many colleagues contributed something, knowingly or unknowingly, to this work. I want to thank in particular, Tom Weil, Steve Hatch, and Hugo Finarelli for their teaching and insights.

Needless to say, I learned quite a bit about strategic planning from my clients over the years. Clients who were generous enough to allow me to include in this text portions of their strategic plans for illustrative purposes include: Pinnacle Health System, Harrisburg, PA; Mission–St. Joseph's Health System, Asheville, NC; Columbia/St. David's Health Care System, Austin, TX; and KidsPeace, Bethlehem, PA. Many other clients educated me, as well, and to all of them, a collective thank you.

Lastly, no work like this can be completed without the support of family and friends. My wife, Rita Bernstein, and children, Seth and Joanna, endured hundreds (thousands?) of hours of complaining, concern, handwringing, and other minutia that are part and parcel of any significant project or work. Thanks for listening and largely saying very little.

Alan M. Zuckerman
Philadelphia, PA
July 1997

Strategic Planning for Healthcare Organizations: Planning Amid Turmoil

NO INDUSTRY in the 1990s has experienced such phenomenal growth and environmental turbulence as the U.S. healthcare delivery system. Since 1980, healthcare expenditures have quadrupled and now represent about 14 percent of the gross domestic product.[1] Factor in the reversal of economic incentives, a technological revolution, regulatory changes, eroding public trust, and government-led reform initiatives with healthcare's exponential growth, and turmoil is the term that best describes what today's healthcare providers are facing.

With the amount and pace of change showing no signs of abating, the greatest challenge facing healthcare managers today is to plan amid the chaos. Pummeled by pressures to reduce costs, improve quality, assume economic risk, and broker affiliations, providers can easily lose sight of strategies needed to position organizations for long-term success, particularly when healthcare has become one of the most complex and dynamic industries in the country. The large number of healthcare organizations that are failing, and the flurry of mergers, acquisitions, and alliances, are indicators of the massive restructuring that is occurring.

Strategic planning is a well-tested approach that is experiencing a resurgence among organizations that must develop forward-looking, feasible strategies, or face potential demise. Healthcare providers have typically been slow to use modern management techniques, such as strategic planning, in favor of maintaining the status quo and weathering environmental changes.[2] But a heightened sense of urgency is emerging for providers who realize they can and must manage their services more efficiently and effectively. The public perception that mismanagement of resources by healthcare organizations has contributed, at least in part, to skyrocketing costs will not be swayed by soft-sell marketing campaigns. And employers, insurance companies, and government agencies are not likely to ease up on their demands for more input into how, where, and by whom healthcare services are provided.

This chapter will define what healthcare strategic planning is, present an overview of the planning process and environment, and discuss why strategic planning is critical to the success of all providers in the twenty-first century.

STRATEGIC PLANNING IS . . .

The concept of strategy has roots in both political and military history, from Sun Tzu to Euripides.[3] The Greek verb *stratego* means "to plan the destruction of one's enemies."[4] Many terms associated with strategic planning, such as objective, mission, strength, and weakness, were developed by or used in the military.[5]

A number of definitions have evolved to pinpoint the essence of strategic planning. According to Duncan, Ginter, and Swayne (1995), "strategic planning is the set of processes used in an organization to understand the situation and develop decision-making guidelines (the strategy) for the organization."[6] Campbell (1993) adds the concept of measurement to his definition: "Strategic planning refers to a process for defining organizational objectives, implementing strategies to achieve those objectives, and measuring the effectiveness of those strategies."[7] Evashwick and Evashwick (1988), including the concepts of vision and mission in their definition, define strategic planning as "the process for assessing a changing environment to create a vision of the future, determining how the organization fits into the anticipated environment based on its institutional mission, strengths, and weaknesses; and then setting in motion a plan of action to position the organization accordingly."[8]

Strategic planning has been used in the business sector for the past 50 years. The concept of planning, programming, and budgeting systems was introduced in the late 1940s and early 1950s and used only sparingly by business and government.[9] In the 1960s and 1970s, leading firms, such as General Electric, practiced strategic planning, promoting the merits of providing a framework beyond the 12-month cycle and a systematic approach to managing business units.[10] Strategic planning in the 1980s and 1990s has been based on corporate market planning, which emphasizes maximizing profits through identification of a market segment and development of strategies to control that segment.[11] Today more than 97 percent of the top 100 industrial companies in the United States report using strategic planning activities.[12]

Strategic planning has been used by healthcare organizations somewhat sporadically since the 1970s, and it has been oriented toward providing services and meeting the needs of the population. Prior to the 1970s, hospitals were predominately independent and not-for-profit, and healthcare planning was usually conducted on a local or regional basis by state, county, or municipal governments. Other elements of the healthcare system were nearly universally far smaller and less organizationally complex than hospitals and, until recently, evidenced little need or desire for formal strategic planning.

The use of strategic planning has waned during recent years with reengineering and total quality management (TQM) rising in popularity as quick fixes for lagging financial performance. While reengineering and TQM are powerful tools for reshaping individual processes, these efforts often overlook how to manage the processes once they have been improved and fail to focus on strategic issues, such as the organization's position in the market. TQM and reengineering also often fail to consider environmental issues, improving a process to compete in an environment that no longer exists.[13]

Cost consciousness takes precedence today. The external and competitive forces that prompted businesses to adopt strategic planning are now being felt full-force by the healthcare industry. Strategic planning must now focus on determining if there is consumer demand for specific services and assessing whether the organization has the resources to provide these services. This broader planning focus, in which market and service information is integrated with financial analyses, must include an openness to buying or brokering products and services, rather than relying on internal development.[14] According to Spiegel and Hyman (1991), "in essence health care providers move from a service-based orientation to a profit-motivated one, from serving a general public regardless of internal needs and profits to a selective population that will guarantee organizational survival through generating profits."[15] Planners must also determine how to work with other providers to survive financially and fulfill the organization's mission.

THE STRATEGIC PLANNING PROCESS

Many variations of a strategic planning model have emerged in both the business and healthcare sectors, but the basic model has remained relatively unchanged since its inception. Two similar versions of strategic planning emerged in the 1980s. Sorkin, Ferris, and Hudak (1984) presented their basic steps of strategic planning:

- scan the environment;
- select key issues;
- set mission statements and broad goals;
- undertake external and internal analyses;
- develop goals, objectives, and strategies for each issue;
- develop an implementation plan to carry out strategic actions; and
- monitor, update, and scan.[16]

Simyar, Lloyd-Jones, and Caro (1988) tailored the process to healthcare strategic planning:

- identify the organization's current position, including present mission, long-term objectives, strategies, and policies;
- analyze the environment;
- conduct an organizational audit;
- identify the various alternative strategies based on relevant data;
- select the best alternative;
- gain acceptance;
- prepare long-range and short-range plans to support and carry out the strategy; and
- implement the plan and conduct an ongoing evaluation.[17]

For the purposes of this book, these various steps of strategic planning have been synthesized into the four stages illustrated in Figure 1.1. The first stage is the situation analysis that focuses on the question of where are we now, and includes four activities:

1. organizational review, including mission, philosophy, and culture;
2. external assessment of the market structure and dynamics;
3. internal assessment of distinctive characteristics; and
4. evaluation of competitive position, including advantages and disadvantages.

The goal of situation analysis is to determine which factors are subject to the organization's control, and how the organization will be affected by external forces.

The second stage of the planning process is strategic direction, followed by the third stage of strategy formulation. Stages two and three address the question, Where should we be going? The main activity of the strategic direction stage is to develop a future strategic

Figure 1.1 Strategic Planning Approach

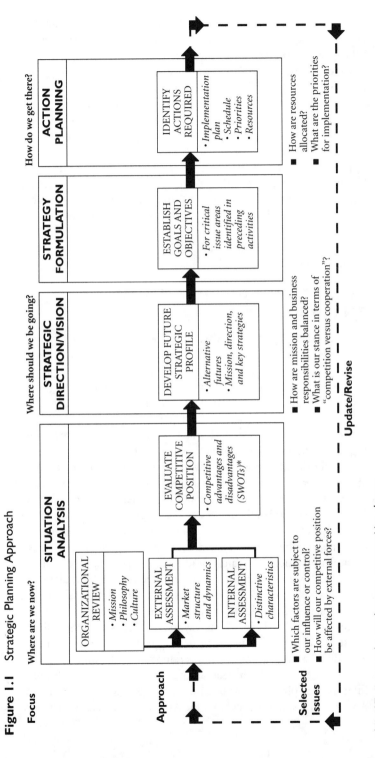

SWOTs = strengths, weaknesses, opportunities, threats.

profile of the organization by examining alternative futures, mission, vision, and key strategies. Strategy formulation, stage three, establishes goals and objectives for the organization. The purpose of these stages of the planning process is to determine what broad, future direction is possible and desirable, and what, generally, the organization is going to target as its future scope of services and position.

The fourth and final stage is action planning, determining how we get there. This stage involves identifying the actions needed to implement the plan. Key activities include setting a schedule, determining priorities, and allocating resources to ensure implementation. While implementation needs to occur as soon as possible after completion of the plan, if not actually during this final stage, a return to the initial stages and updating of the plan, at least in part, ensures that strategic planning becomes an ongoing activity of the organization. Each of these stages will be discussed in detail in the following chapters.

THE STRATEGIC PLANNING ENVIRONMENT

While the definitions of strategic planning may seem relatively basic and straightforward and the process a clear-cut sequence of activities, effective strategic planning is an intricate process of self-examination, forecasting the future, fleshing out problems and determining solutions, choosing a course of action into potentially unknown territory, and then bringing the plan to life. The process becomes even more daunting considering the past influences that have shaped healthcare organizations and the pressures that lie ahead.

Other than technological advances, the most sweeping changes affecting healthcare organizations have been in the payment environment. Since 1966, four phases of the payment environment have emerged.[18] The end of the 1960s was a calm, prosperous environment for healthcare organizations with an abundant fee-for-service and cost-plus-reimbursement system. During this "entitlement" phase, as implementation of Medicare and Medicaid generated surging demand, healthcare organizations had little need for strategic planning.

From 1972 to 1982, the payment system was relatively stable, but some strategy was needed to maximize reimbursement and create cost reports that justified expenses to payors. This "growth without limit" phase found providers playing catch up as the increasing demand exceeded the supply. The result was rampaging inflation.

By the mid-1980s, the federal government's 20-year involvement in healthcare planning was rescinded. President Ronald Reagan, the American Hospital Association, the American Medical Association, and others claimed that stimulating competition, rather than relying on federal regulation, would more effectively contain medical costs. A prospective payment system using diagnosis-related groups (DRGs) for reimbursement, the proliferation of managed care, and the shift of much inpatient care to the ambulatory setting were viewed as more promising alternatives for holding down costs than reliance on certificate-of-need and rate regulation.[19] During this period, proprietary providers emerged as a significant influence in healthcare delivery, taking advantage of unrestrained growth in demand and considerable potential for profitability brought on by DRGs and scale economy opportunities.

The past ten years have undoubtedly been the most turbulent for the healthcare industry. The prospective payment system has shifted providers' mindsets from quality healthcare at any cost to cost containment. The proliferation of managed care systems such as preferred provider organizations (PPOs) and health maintenance organizations (HMOs) has spurred growth of integrated healthcare delivery. These developments, along with peer review organizations that serve as quality and utilization watchdogs, have fueled a competitive environment in which many healthcare organizations find themselves in a tailspin.

Regulation, competition, and the consolidated purchasing power of public and private payors have resulted in what many people are labeling "bare bones" reimbursement. Healthcare organization incomes have been dropping due to lower reimbursement, decreasing demand in some sectors, and high fixed costs. As healthcare organizations lose patient volume, the losses come directly off the bottom line because costs do not drop in proportion to lower admissions. A 1993 survey by the Healthcare Financial Management Association attests to the pressures facing hospital executives. According to 32 percent of survey respondents, declining margins is the most significant challenge facing chief executive officers (CEOs) of hospitals.[20]

Trends for the Future

The future healthcare environment shows no signs of being "kinder and gentler" to providers. A number of trends on the horizon will affect providers and their decisions about the future.

Providers will assume increasing risk for underutilization and overutilization of services.

Economic risk is shifting from insurance companies and employers to providers. Comprehensive systems will assume risk for a defined population group, and will be paid a fixed fee per covered life. By keeping the group of covered lives healthy, and providing and controlling a full continuum of services for their patients, providers will reduce utilization and, ultimately, costs. The philosophical shift from building volume by increasing admissions, tests, and procedures, to keeping a population healthy and reducing utilization will not come easily.

Only unique or geographically isolated providers will remain independent.

Providers in the healthcare system of the future will be closely aligned. Partnerships, alliances, mergers, and consolidations are the watchwords for healthcare providers of the future. Adversarial relationships will lead to failure.

Healthcare reform is occurring parallel to, and in spite of, state and federal healthcare reform initiatives.

Universal insurance coverage, healthcare purchasing groups, and other reform measures may eventually develop. In the meantime, many providers are reforming themselves. Legislation may simply formalize changes already occurring.

Technological advances will enhance and challenge healthcare delivery.

Existing and developing technology has enormous potential to improve efficiency and productivity, but often at a high price. Use of technology may increase operational costs and drain resources if the value of the technology is not proven to reduce staffing or resource utilization.

Providers must manage excess capacity.

As inpatient and specialist utilization continues to drop and many services move beyond the traditional institutional setting, providers must cope with the burden of excess capacity. Consolidating or closing down services and reallocating resources to provide services that maintain or improve economic viability are imperatives facing providers.

Limitations on reimbursement for high-cost services will stimulate continued growth of ambulatory care services and increase demand for post-acute options.

With continued emphasis on cost containment, providing services on an outpatient basis will be a viable, cost-saving option for providers.

Home healthcare, skilled nursing centers, and rehabilitation facilities will help healthcare organizations downstage patients out of costly acute care settings. Primary care, including dramatically increased use of physician extenders, will continue as a substitute for specialty medical services.

As healthcare moves toward an all managed care system, the number of physicians needed will drop dramatically resulting in an oversupply of physicians, particularly specialists.

The oversupply of physicians may have lasting effects on the quality, availability, and costs of healthcare. Options for physicians include planning early retirement, practicing in underserved communities, and seeking retraining as primary care physicians.

WHY STRATEGIC PLANNING?

With the chaos pervading the healthcare field, many executives and not-for-profit boards may wonder if it is possible to plan effectively or plan at all given the uncertainty ahead. Indeed, many providers are *not* conducting comprehensive strategic planning. Research shows that many providers fail to evaluate the environment in which they operate. A study by Zallocco and Joseph (1991) evaluated 13 activities considered to be a part of strategic market planning.[21] The three activities categorized as environmental analysis (market analysis, competitive analysis, and general consumer surveys) were performed by less than half of the hospitals surveyed.

Many healthcare organizations that have undertaken strategic planning experienced problems that jaded their leaders to the value of planning. Several problems are typically encountered during the strategic planning process.

Failing to involve the appropriate people in the process

The CEO typically serves as the strategic leader while development and selection of the strategy is the role of line managers who must bring the plan to life. Involvement of physician and community leaders is also essential to ensure widespread support for the plan.

Conducting strategic planning independently of financial planning

If financial considerations are excluded from the strategic plan, strategies may never become a reality. Sound strategic planning will include financial screening of strategic options.

Failing to develop consensus on the organization's internal and external environment

Planning participants will become polarized if agreement is not reached on the current position of the organization and the existing and future operating environment.

Falling prey to paralysis of analysis

The fast-paced healthcare market demands that providers respond to opportunities and threats without extensive delays. Many providers are lulled into a sense of security when they are planning and squander time over endless fine-tuning and revisions. When exhaustive planning takes over, very little change or progress occurs.

Not addressing the critical issues

The most pressing issues may not be addressed because the board and other planning participants assume the organization's leaders are handling these problems. If no one is prepared to initiate discussions of key issues, strategic plans focus on minor topics and ignore the most critical and threatening ones.

Assuming that once objectives are established they will take care of themselves

Failure to implement a strategic plan is one of the most common flaws of the planning process. Staff may be overwhelmed with managing day-to-day crises, leaving little time to implement strategic objectives. The objectives may also lack precision, so that ensuing activities lack direction.

So why should providers conduct comprehensive strategic planning? Why not rely on ad hoc planning based on educated guesses and intuition? Healthcare organizations may have historically survived using less formalized approaches to make policy decisions, but today's providers must be more precise in their choices. Mistakes will not only result in lost revenue, but closure.

There are many tangible benefits of strategic planning that continue long after the plan is completed. Duncan, Ginter and Swayne (1995) identified the following benefits of strategic planning.[22]

- may improve financial performance;
- provides the organization with self-concept, specific goals, guidance, and consistency of decision making;
- encourages managers to understand the present, plan for the future, and understand when change is vital;
- requires managers to communicate vertically and horizontally;
- improves overall coordination within the organization; and

- encourages innovation and change to meet the challenges of a complex and evolving environment.

According to Nadler (1994), for many organizations the true value lies in the planning process, not the plan. "Most plans have a tremendously fast rate of depreciation. By the time they're printed and bound they've become obsolete. The value of planning is largely in the shared learning, the shared frame of reference, the shared context for those small decisions that get made over time."[23] Indeed changes may occur daily that influence a strategic plan, and new ideas may surface once the plan is complete. A successful strategic plan enables providers to establish a consistent, articulated direction for the future. But it is also a living document that must be monitored and revised to meet both anticipated and unanticipated needs of the organization and the market, whether these changes are related to managed care, integrated delivery, healthcare reform, systems development, technological advances, or other challenges on the horizon.

Notes

1. Bureau of the Census. 1995. *Statistical Abstract of the United States.* Washington, D.C.
2. Duncan, W. J., P. M. Ginter, and L. E. Swayne. 1995. *Strategic Management of Health Care Organizations.* Boston: PWS-Kent Publishing Company, p. 17.
3. Ibid.
4. Bracker, J. 1980. "The Historical Development of the Strategic Management Concept." *Academy of Management Review* 5 (2): 219–24.
5. Duncan, Ginter, and Swayne.
6. Ibid.
7. Campbell, A. B. 1993. "Strategic Planning in Health Care: Methods and Applications." *Quality Management in Health Care* 1 (4): 13.
8. Evashwick, C. J., and W. T. Evashwick. 1988. "The Fine Art of Strategic Planning." *Provider* 14 (4): 4–6.
9. Webster, J. L., W. R. Reif, and J. S. Bracker. 1989. "The Manager's Guide to Strategic Planning Tools and Techniques." *Planning Review* 17 (6): 5.
10. Ibid.
11. Spiegel, A. D., and H. H. Hyman. 1991. *Strategic Health Planning: Methods and Techniques Applied to Marketing and Management.* Norwood, NJ: Ablex Publishing Corporation.
12. Klein, H. E., and R. E. Linneman. 1984. "Environmental Assessment: An International Study of Corporate Practice." *The Journal of Business Strategy* 5, 66–75.
13. Garvin, D. A. 1995. "Leveraging Processes for Strategic Advantage." *Harvard Business Review* 73 (5): 80.
14. Goldman, E. F., and K. C. Nolan. 1994. *Strategic Planning in Health Care: A Guide for Board Members.* Chicago: American Hospital Publishing, Inc.
15. Spiegel and Hyman, p. 8.

16. Sorkin, D. L., N. B. Ferris, and J. Hudak. 1984. "Strategies for Cities and Counties." In *A Strategic Planning Guide*. Washington, D.C.: Public Technology, Inc.

17. Simyar, F., J. Lloyd-Jones, and J. Caro. 1988. "Strategic Management: A Proposed Framework for the Health Care Industry." In *Strategic Management in the Health Care Sector: Toward the Year 2000*, edited by F. Simyar and J. Lloyd-Jones, 6–17. Englewood Cliffs, NJ: Prentice Hall.

18. Eastaugh, S. R. 1992. "Hospital Strategy and Financial Performance." *Health Care Management Review* 17 (3): 20.

19. Spiegel and Hyman.

20. Cerne, F. 1993. "Strategic Shakeup." *Hospitals* 67 (7): 28.

21. Zallocco, R. L., and W. B. Joseph. 1991. "Strategic Market Planning in Hospitals: Is It Done? Does It Work?" *Journal of Health Care Marketing* 11 (1): 5–11.

22. Duncan, Ginter, and Swayne, p. 9.

23. Nadler, D. A. 1994. "Collaborative Strategic Thinking." *Planning Review* 22 (5): 30.

CHAPTER *2*

Organizing for Successful Strategic Planning: Ten Critical Steps

I T IS TELLING that in drafting and redrafting an outline for this book, and then beginning the actual writing of it, this chapter was omitted. Like many in the field, I chose instead to plunge in to performing the actual work and began to describe the process and product of strategic planning. However, as I tried to describe what must be accomplished in strategic planning and why, I realized I had left out the most critical first activity, organizing for successful strategic planning.

Why was a chapter on organizing not conceptualized as part of this book originally or even well into the writing of the first draft? On reflection, I suspect it is the bias toward action that most of us have. Also, organizing seems boring and obvious to many and drudge work to nearly all.

Yet, as I reflect on the hundreds of strategic plans I have reviewed, and the many planning and management staffs I have spoken with about strategic planning, it is clear that one of the common mistakes in an organization's strategic planning process is the failure to organize before the "work" of strategic planning begins. To correct this problem, the following ten steps are critical to carry out in advance of strategic planning to ensure successful initiation of the planning process:

1. Identify and communicate strategic planning objectives.

2. Describe and communicate the planning process.

3. Define and communicate roles and responsibilities of organization leadership.
4. Plan and communicate the strategic planning schedule.
5. Assemble relevant historical data.
6. Resolve not to overanalyze historical data.
7. Review past strategies and identify successes and failures.
8. Conduct strategic planning orientation meeting.
9. Prepare to stimulate "new thinking."
10. Reinforce future orientation.

Identify and Communicate Strategic Planning Objectives

The word "communicate" is integral to the first four steps of organizing for strategic planning. One of the failures of healthcare strategic planning in the recent past is too much analysis by too few. To be successful, the process needs to include as many elements of organization leadership as possible and as many different perspectives as possible. To ensure that widespread participation occurs in the planning process, the organizational phase of the strategic planning process needs to emphasize communication of strategic planning objectives.

The importance of clear objectives in successful strategic planning cannot be overemphasized. While some may find it satisfactory to state as an objective that "strategic planning will provide our organization with a road map for the future," or "strategic planning will allow our organization to allocate scarce resources in the most effective manner possible," these general strategic planning objectives are probably not specific enough to prove to all constituencies that it is worthwhile to expend the time and resources required for strategic planning. More specific strategic planning objectives should be established and reviewed periodically during the strategic planning process to ensure that the process is addressing priority issues and that the plan is on track to produce outputs that satisfy these objectives.

Although there is a wide range of potential objectives a healthcare organization may establish for its strategic plan, some of the more specific objectives for the healthcare delivery environment of the late 1990s have included determining:

- whether to remain a freestanding entity;
- how to respond to decreasing reimbursement per unit of service provided;
- whether to or how to develop and offer an integrated continuum of care; and
- how to position for managed care.

It is the role of senior management to clearly define these or other objectives for the strategic planning process; review them with board leadership, physicians, and other important stakeholders; and communicate them broadly and regularly to the organization during the strategic planning process.

Describe and Communicate the Planning Process

There is an abundance of material on strategic planning processes and approaches for healthcare organizations to draw on. A well-tested strategic planning process, adapted for the current healthcare delivery environment, is described in detail throughout this book. Case studies are included to illustrate how the process may be tailored for different healthcare organizations. The preceding chapter provided a brief summary of recent healthcare and business strategic planning literature with references to a variety of texts on contemporary strategic planning. Whether the strategic process described in this book is selected, or one from another source is chosen, it is imperative to select a planning process and customize it to meet the organization's specific needs prior to initiating strategic planning.

Too often, planning begins without a clear sense of what the planning process entails. In these cases, planning often commences as a reaction to strategic planning questions raised by the board or senior management. As the questions are being answered, management decides that the questions are best answered within the context of a yet unspecified strategic planning process. Thus, migration into what is called strategic planning begins without a careful and thoughtful attempt to understand why or how strategic planning should occur.

Once a strategic planning process is developed to meet the specific strategic planning objectives of the organization, this process must be communicated effectively to organization leadership and other important stakeholders. Without an understanding of the planning process, leadership and stakeholders will feel removed from the strategic planning and reluctant to participate or participate ineffectively.

Define and Communicate Roles and Responsibilities of Organization Leadership

Strategic planning is one of the major responsibilities of executive management. It is also an important activity of the board, with its role of advisor on policy to management. In healthcare organizations, strategic planning is also a mechanism to bring physicians, who usually are not employed by the organization, into the process of collectively determining what direction should be taken in the future, both for the healthcare organization itself and indirectly for related entities such as physician groups.

There is substantial diversity of opinion in the literature as to the importance of and the breadth and depth of involvement of key organization constituencies in the planning process. Some believe that strategic planning is principally the responsibility of executive management and that participation of other elements of the organization in the planning process should be limited. Others believe that the best plans are developed if there is broad and frequent participation by all key stakeholders in the organization. The perspective espoused in this book, while neither of these extremes, is somewhat closer to the latter view. Chapter 7 further discusses this issue.

Here, as in the previous two planning preparation steps, there is no single answer for every organization, but rather a choice to be made from among available alternatives. Regardless of the level of participation selected, the decision, typically made by senior management, should be made before the planning process actually begins and communicated clearly to all affected constituencies. Once the strategic planning process is formally initiated, board members, management staff, physicians, and others will then understand their roles in the planning process and what specific responsibilities they will have as the planning process unfolds.

Plan and Communicate the Strategic Planning Schedule

Although strategic planning should be an ongoing activity of every organization, it is necessary to carry out a full strategic plan development process or update a current plan every three to five years. Most organizations that practice ongoing strategic planning have annual planning cycles and schedules. In such situations, a full strategic plan development process is also carried out in 12 months or less.

There is a diversity of opinion among strategic planning experts about the optimal duration of the full strategic planning process. Some believe it is best to complete the plan as quickly as possible to maintain a high degree of focus on the planning process during its duration. Others believe that a more extended schedule is better, allowing for broader participation and reflection on planning analyses and intermediate outputs during the process.

This book takes a perspective that is between these two extremes, although it is generally closer to the latter view. Here again there is a choice to be made by senior management among available alternatives, with related pros and cons. As with the previous three steps, the choice should be made deliberately and consciously, in advance of the initiation of planning activities and clearly communicated to all affected constituencies.

Assemble Relevant Historical Data

Accurate and complete data are an asset to strategic planning. Conversely, the lack of accurate and complete data can be a major impediment to the strategic plan.

It is never too early to assemble a historical database for strategic planning. Data profiling the past three to five years of the organization's performance and of the market in which it operates should be compiled and routinely updated. The specific types of data required and analytical approaches will be discussed in Chapter 3. The main point here is twofold: (1) to stress the importance of an early start on the time-consuming data collection process, which is often difficult to complete in a reasonable time frame; and (2) to emphasize that it is critical to devote ample time and effort to the task of data collection to ensure an accurate and complete database.

Often, analyses are conducted only to discover partway through the process or as the results are being reviewed that essential data are, in fact, missing or that the data are, in part, inaccurate. This is discouraging at a minimum and disabling at worst, especially if the problem is discovered in a public forum and undermines the credibility of the strategic planning process. Getting an early start on assembling the historical database and building in adequate time for review and validation of accuracy and completeness of the data is an indispensable, yet infrequently used, approach to ensure high-quality strategic planning.

Resolve Not to Overanalyze Historical Data

Historical data assembled to aid strategic planning can be a great asset, but it can also be a trap into which the organization falls. Two major pitfalls can occur to hinder serious strategic planning.

Inability to assemble the required database

It is clearly a subjective decision as to how much historical data are required for sound planning. There are frequently a few members of the planning team who want more or better data, and will disable the planning process before it begins or derail it through a series of challenges to its validity.

Undue focus on analyses of past performance

A related problem is the penchant for planning team members to analyze every facet of historical performance. More analyses can always be carried out. The decision about the scope and extent of historical data analysis is a subjective one, and every effort should be made in advance to determine what analyses are necessary for sound strategic planning to limit lengthy delays.

Although it can be comforting to focus on the past and dwell on the known rather than the unknown, strategic planning is primarily focused on preparing to deal with the future. There is clear value in understanding past successes and failures, but organizations should resolve to use historical data for its intended purpose of guiding future forecasts and strategies.

Review Past Strategies and Identify Successes and Failures

Part of the important historical analysis that must be completed is a review of the organization's past strategies, its successes, and its failures. This activity is often best completed in advance of formal commencement of the strategic planning process for three reasons: (1) it will help determine how best to structure the strategic planning process itself; (2) it will highlight certain types of analyses that may be important to successful planning in a particular situation; and (3) it will identify issues that the organization must be aware of as it formulates its new strategies and implementation approaches.

An objective review of past strategies can be very revealing. Often the actual strategies used by an organization are quite different from those that may have been proposed in a previous strategic plan. Similarly, the actual strategies employed by the organization may vary to some degree from those that organization leadership perceives were being followed. A review of historical documents by someone outside the inner circle, either a new senior staff member or a consultant, and a discussion of what was proposed, perceived, and actually occurred over the past three to five years can be a fascinating and important pre-planning process exercise.

As part of this process, it is also important to review what has worked, what has not, and why. Often, inadequate attention is paid in formal planning to failed strategies, which can lead to reoccurring mistakes. Thorough, honest evaluation of successful and unsuccessful strategies can help an organization avoid this common pitfall.

Conduct Strategic Planning Orientation Meetings

The first formal step in the initiation of the strategic planning process is to conduct one or more strategic planning orientation meetings. These meetings should be scheduled and held during the pre-planning stage.

In most healthcare organizations, a strategic planning committee is established as the focal point for oversight of the strategic planning process. This committee may be a standing committee of the board or created to serve on an ad hoc basis. This committee should have its initial orientation meeting during this phase. This project initiation session should aim to:

- describe and discuss strategic planning objectives;
- review and revise the strategic planning approach and schedule, including identification of key project meetings and other milestones;
- review the initial database and identify sources for any additional data required;
- identify internal and external interviewees;
- identify other primary market research to be conducted, including intended audiences and purpose of market research; and
- discuss the mechanisms for interface among the planning staff, consultants (as applicable), and the organization including:
  - structure of the strategic planning steering committee;
  - staff contacts for logistical support;
  - interaction with the board, medical staff, and other constituents; and
  - logistical issues related to the project.

As part of engagement initiation, a planning retreat may be held with senior management and the strategic planning steering committee. The purpose of this retreat may be to review the organization's past planning initiatives, including successes and failures; identify and explore important environmental trends and potential impacts; and discuss key planning issues already defined, including potential alternatives to address these issues.

It may be desirable to convene strategic planning orientation sessions for various other groups in the organization at this point. Depending on the size and complexity of the organization and decisions about the breadth and depth of participation sought in the strategic planning process, orientation sessions may be held with the board in its entirety, other members of the senior management staff, physicians, other professional staff, or occasionally municipal government leaders or community groups. These orientation sessions will usually focus on just a few of the areas outlined, such as objectives for strategic planning, planning process and schedule, and future role of the affected constituencies in the planning process.

Prepare to Stimulate "New Thinking"

As previously discussed, it is easy to get caught up in analyzing the past and never engage in true strategic planning. There is a temptation to extrapolate, literally and figuratively, from the performances and experiences of the past and devise future strategy on this premise. In the more orderly and less frenetic world of past decades, good planning strategy may have resulted from this approach. But with rapid and nonlinear changes occurring at an ever-faster pace, this type of thinking is likely to lead to naive strategies at best.

Another problem-laden strategic planning method frequently used by healthcare organizations is adopting or mimicking known strategies used by other organizations in demographically similar, but more advanced regional markets. This practice usually takes the form of midwestern or eastern organizations studying what is occurring in California or a similar advanced market in order to understand and adapt the already successful methods. Although this approach may work, it is not without significant pitfalls, including lack of comparability of seemingly similar situations and failure to understand the actual strategy and plan in the more advanced market.

While we certainly can and should learn from others in similar situations, it is at least equally important to try to break new ground and be innovative with plans and strategies. As described in subsequent chapters, healthcare planners need to be much more thoughtful and creative about describing the future environment, understanding implications of changing environmental conditions, and considering potential strategies that enable organizations to realize their objectives. Much of the strategic planning by healthcare organizations assumes a static competitive environment. This approach is at odds with today's reality and will be increasingly inconsistent with the more dynamic era we are entering.

There is an enormous body of literature on techniques and approaches for stimulating more creative thinking—a list of suggested readings is presented at the end of this chapter. Preparation for the strategic planning process in each organization should include a review of literature, consideration of organization needs and potential alternative processes, and selection of techniques that may help the organization leap forward in its strategic development.

Reinforce Future Orientation

To successfully plan for the future, healthcare organizations require a new perspective on the future. This perspective needs to be broader, bolder, and more creative and dynamic. To counter the tendency to overemphasize the past and present circumstances, organization leaders need to overcompensate and continually push their organizations to break with the past and consider alternative futures that are very different from today's known circumstances. Injecting this kind of thinking into healthcare strategic planning will invigorate the process and lead to much more thoughtful plans and strategies. These are the plans and strategies that will set the new standard by which successful planning and development is measured early in the twenty-first century.

Healthcare strategic planning is at a relatively immature stage in its developmental process. Within this chapter alone, healthcare strategic planning has been characterized as historically focused, lacking creativity, preoccupied with mimicry, haphazardly applied, poorly planned for, and so forth. Part of the problem is due to a lack of clear, meaningful objectives, and part also is a function of the failure to adequately prepare to plan, both by staff and other important members of the organization. This chapter has addressed both of these deficits and hopefully will heighten awareness of the need to prepare and adequately carry out successful strategic planning.

Suggested Readings

Brightman, H. J. 1980. *Problem Solving: A Logical and Creative Approach.* Atlanta, GA: Business Publishing Division, Georgia State University.

de Bono, E. 1992. *Serious Creativity.* New York: Harper Collins Publishers, Inc.

————. 1994. *Parallel Thinking.* New York: Penguin Books U.S.A., Inc.

Garrat, B. (ed.). 1995. *Developing Strategic Thought.* New York: McGraw-Hill Book Company.

Michalko, M. 1991. *Thinkertoys.* Berkeley, CA: Ten Speed Press.

Parnes, S. J. (ed.). 1992. *Source Book for Creative Problem-Solving.* Buffalo, NY: Creative Education Foundation Press.

Prather, C. W., and L. K. Gundry. 1995. *Blueprints for Innovation.* New York: AMA Membership Publications Division.

Runco, M. A. 1994. *Problem Finding, Problem Solving, and Creativity.* Norwood, NJ: Ablex Publishing Corporation.

CHAPTER 3

Activity I: Analyzing the Situation

LOOKING FORWARD VS. LOOKING BACKWARD

STRATEGIC PLANNING typically begins with an analysis of the current and recent situation of the organization. This activity is referred to as the situation analysis or environmental assessment.

In many ways the situation analysis sets the tone for the strategic plan. As the first activity in the planning process, it provides an indication of how the rest of the planning process is likely to unfold.

- Will the process be comprehensive in scope?
- Will the process constructively involve key organization stakeholders?
- Will the process be highly structured or loosely organized?
- Have the objectives of the strategic planning process been clearly articulated, and will they be followed?
- Is a planning schedule being followed, and can it be anticipated that planning will lead to action in the foreseeable future?

Many planning efforts get off to poor starts because the planning process and activities have been insufficiently conceptualized in advance, not well organized, or inadequately communicated to all elements of the organization at the outset, as discussed in Chapter 2. A second and equally serious problem is the tendency for staff to become enmeshed in data gathering and analysis bogging down the planning process early on in "analysis paralysis." While it is important to compile a database that clearly reflects the organization's historical performance and the market in which it has operated, strategic planning is not primarily an exercise in plotting historical patterns and then extrapolating forward. There is comfort in looking back over recent history and analyzing successes and failures and, unlike other aspects of strategic planning, it is at least theoretically possible to compile an unequivocally accurate picture, albeit of the past. However, there is little to be gained from overanalysis of the past and whatever momentum and excitement the organization may be able to create at the initiation of strategic planning is likely to be lost if historical performance becomes the major focus of the strategic planning process.

APPROACH TO THE INTERNAL ASSESSMENT

The internal assessment combines data analysis and qualitative information to formulate an accurate profile of the historical performance of the organization. Along with the external assessment, it profiles the organization's strengths, weaknesses, opportunities, and threats (SWOTs), and identifies competitive advantages and disadvantages that serve as a springboard to subsequent strategic planning activities. There are five main components of the internal assessment.

Review role statements and organizational framework.

This activity is a high-level review to determine whether the organization does as it says it will do, and has an organizational structure and processes that allow it to achieve its objectives. The review includes an assessment of current mission, vision, and values statements and compares them to recent performance. Current and recent changes in organization structure and processes are also compared to program development and financial performance.

Analyze characteristics and utilization trends of the overall organization, its component entities, and their programs and services.

Although organizations are often tempted to profile all programs and services in this task, it rarely makes sense to profile more than the top 75 to 80 percent of all programs and services individually (as measured by volume or financial contribution), though all or nearly all should be inventoried. The profile of programs and services should include capacity, volumes, and key resource attributes for the past three to five years.

Conduct primary market research.

There are two primary purposes of market research: (1) to gather pertinent information on the strengths and weaknesses of the organization and its competitors in the marketplace; and (2) to involve organization leadership constructively and broadly early in the strategic planning process. This activity should begin with a review of any recent (one to three years) primary market research. Then additional research can be initiated, including personal interviews, focus groups, written surveys, or telephone surveys. Research targets typically include board members, physicians, other health professionals, and upper and middle management staff. This task, when performed well, has almost limitless returns. Although the substantive value of the market research often diminishes significantly with greater and greater amounts of research, the political value of soliciting and carefully listening to opinions of organization leaders cannot be overestimated. The researchers must clearly indicate at the outset, however, that they are listening through note taking and feedback following research.

Analyze other critical resources.

This task generally focuses on facilities, equipment, and staff to identify major assets and liabilities. Comparison to industry norms and competitors in the local marketplace is appropriate.

Analyze financial performance and position.

Financial performance for the entire organization and its major component entities for the past three to five years should be profiled and compared to industry norms and competitors in the local marketplace. If the organization has already prepared future financial projections for the next one to three years, these should be included in the analysis.

The product of the internal assessment should be a maximum of 20 charts or tables, except for the largest and most complex healthcare organizations that may need additional analysis, with modest narration or highlighting of key points. While three to five times as many analytical tables and other supporting documents may be prepared and available as back-up, there is no reason why the internal assessment report cannot be shortened for ease of understanding and use.

APPROACH TO THE EXTERNAL
ASSESSMENT

The external assessment, like the internal assessment, combines data analysis and qualitative information to formulate an accurate profile of the historical performance of the organization with reference specifically to the marketplace in which it operates. The external assessment also provides a profile of the historical performance of the marketplace and starts the process of beginning to look forward through its explicit consideration of market trends and forecasts. Listed below are the five main components of the external assessment, with comments on the important analytic underpinnings of each.

Review demographic, economic, and health status trends and forecasts.

Organizations should exercise extreme caution with this activity, since the extent of the analysis often exceeds all reason. It is important to profile key indicators for the past three to five years, and provide forecasts for the next five to ten years, if available. However, the objective of this task is to identify the broadest trends and variables that have had and will have an impact on organization performance. Minor shifts in population, economic performance, or health status are of minimal or no consequence to the strategic planning process. This analysis is occasionally useful in identifying geographic areas or population segments with strong potential for future market penetration.

Review healthcare technology, delivery, reimbursement, and regulatory trends.

The purpose of this task is to identify any major environmental influences, largely occurring at the state or national level, that have affected and will affect the future performance of the organization. Major trends in each category should be profiled for the past three to five years. Forecasts, including potential alternative scenarios, for the next three to five years should be identified and discussed.

Analyze competitors.

This is the most important and often the most difficult task to complete well in the situation analysis. Competitor data in healthcare is usually incomplete and out of date even when available. Of all the situation analysis tasks, by far the most effort and the greatest importance should be assigned to this task. Competitors may exist on a variety of levels. Some organizations may compete in most or all service categories, while other competitors may operate in one or a few selected niches. To profile competitors, data should be collected from regional, state, and national sources. Qualitative information should be gathered from internal and external market research.

Conduct primary market research.

This task parallels the market research activity described in the internal assessment, but focuses on parties external to the organization. The purpose of market research is to gather pertinent information on the position of the organization in its marketplace relative to its competitors. Recent (one to three years) primary market research should be reviewed before proceeding with this task. Market research that may be appropriate includes personal interviews, focus groups, written surveys, or telephone surveys. Targets of research typically include senior managers of competitors, other persons knowledgeable about the healthcare delivery system, and community leaders.

Assess market forecasts and implications.

In some instances, market forecasts may already exist, and should be gathered and assessed. Typically, population changes, economic indicators, and healthcare delivery–specific parameters may already have been the subject of publicly available forecasts. In other cases, forecasts will need to be prepared. At a minimum, projections should use appropriate forecasting techniques for major health service components, including acute, post-acute, and ambulatory care services by major service lines. A list of publications addressing forecasting techniques is presented at the end of this chapter.

A summary of the market structure and dynamics should be prepared parallel to the internal assessment summary. A brief report with no more than 20 charts and tables with modest narration or highlighting of key points and back-up should suffice.

COMPETITIVE ADVANTAGES
AND DISADVANTAGES

The internal and external assessments need to produce two main outputs to facilitate the strategic planning process: a succinct and honest statement of the organization's competitive advantages and disadvantages in the marketplace and an appraisal of key planning issues requiring resolution in the strategic planning process.

There are no universally accepted approaches or formats for determining and displaying competitive advantages and disadvantages. In general, the two most reliable measures of competitive advantage or disadvantage are marketshare and operating margin. Upward historical trends in these variables are usually indicative of strong competitive position. However, the trends evidenced in healthcare organizations are rarely this clear-cut and consistent across multiple services. Occasionally, this simplistic perspective masks major shifts in competitive position occurring as a result of the lagged effect of capital or human investments.

The two most commonly used formats for displaying competitive advantage and disadvantage are the SWOTs summary and a straightforward enumeration of competitive advantages and disadvantages. Examples of the typical outputs of each are shown in

Figures 3.1 and 3.2. While a lengthy listing of SWOTs or competitive advantages and disadvantages may initially be generated, it is desirable to refine the list so that a one-page summary is prepared. As the examples show, items may be drawn from each of the categories of the internal and external assessments already prepared, but not every category needs to be represented in the final summary. The objective of this analysis is to provide organization leadership with a clear assessment of where the organization stands in its competitive marketplace. Little benefit is derived from overly complicating the results. The competitive assessment is a device to assist in determining what planning issues the organization must grapple with in its future development, but is not an end in and of itself.

Two other more quantitative formats have recently been developed and have proven to be useful in determining competitive advantages and disadvantages. Traditionally, competitive analysis in healthcare has focused on the past and the examples cited above are reasonably representative of this. Even when looking forward, competitive analysis has had a fairly static perspective, assuming changes in the market but not in competitor strategies and initiatives. To begin to address this deficit, future-oriented market sizing and modeling and companion modeling of organization performance versus best practices and benchmarks may prove useful.

Figure 3.1   General Hospital Strategic Profile

Strengths
- Geographic location
- Recent operating performance
- Geriatric services
- Relatively high occupancy
- PHO* ahead of the market

Weaknesses
- Relationship to inner city
- Lack of distinctive services
- Obstetrics, Pediatrics, and Emergency Department
- Medical staff (e.g., age, solo, perceived quality)
- Lack of capital reserves
- Declining volumes
- Low case-mix index
- No national affiliation
- Freestanding community hospital

Opportunities
- Increased penetration in core service area
- Network/affiliation arrangement
- Expense and ALOS* reduction
- Increased board effectiveness
- Hospital-physician coordination
- Medical staff development
- Nonacute service development

Threats
- Exclusion from managed care contracts
- Shrinking acute care market
- Forced to remain freestanding
- Increasingly constrained reimbursement

*ALOS—average length of stay; PHO—physician-hospital organization.

Figure 3.2   Rural Healthcare System Competitive Analysis

Competitive Advantages
- Dominant provider in a 15-county region
- Strong financial performance and position
- Marketshare growing
- Viewed as the quality provider
- Competitive costs and prices

Competitive Disadvantages
- Complacent
- Large, cumbersome, and bureaucratic
- Losing share at periphery of region
- Strong competitors outside the region are moving in

Figure 3.3 presents an example macro-level market sizing and share model. The model depicts the amount of healthcare service demands or capacity requirements for a population base of a certain size. It models requirements based on population changes and demand and capacity levels for alternative managed care penetration scenarios. Changing the population base or composition or providing different managed care penetration scenarios will alter the resulting market and capacity sizes. Projected marketshare by service is depicted by the shaded area in the diagram. Alternative marketshare configurations can be generated based on varying assumptions about competitive market dynamics. More service and micro-level analyses can be prepared to account for the service composition and mix of any healthcare provider organization.

The macro-level market sizing and share model, by its nature, is future oriented, can readily factor in different competitive scenario assumptions, and is a great improvement over more qualitative and less rigorous approaches.

Table 3.1 presents an example of an approach to modeling key organization and market characteristics using best practices and benchmarking as a guide to future competitive needs. This approach involves selecting a limited number of important indicators, anywhere from 5 to 15, and modeling organization performance and market requirements based on existing best practices from more advanced markets, assuming the existence of more advanced markets. A target level is then selected based on the analyst's perspective of the likely evolution of the healthcare marketplace. The target may be equal to today's best practice, exceed it (if best practice is likely to evolve to a better practice in the future), or fall short of it (if the affected market may not advance to the competitive dynamics of today's best practice market). Comparing the current organization or

Figure 3.3 Population-Based Demand, Year 2000 for ABC Health System's Service Area, Weighted Managed Care—625,000 Lives

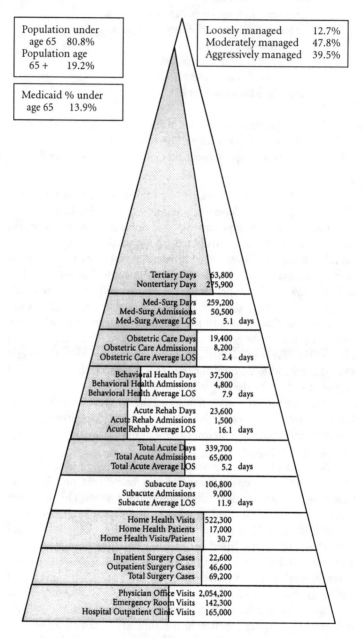

| Population under age 65 | 80.8% |
| Population age 65 + | 19.2% |

| Medicaid % under age 65 | 13.9% |

Loosely managed	12.7%
Moderately managed	47.8%
Aggressively managed	39.5%

Tertiary Days	63,800	
Nontertiary Days	275,900	
Med-Surg Days	259,200	
Med-Surg Admissions	50,500	
Med-Surg Average LOS	5.1	days
Obstetric Care Days	19,400	
Obstetric Care Admissions	8,200	
Obstetric Care Average LOS	2.4	days
Behavioral Health Days	37,500	
Behavioral Health Admissions	4,800	
Behavioral Health Average LOS	7.9	days
Acute Rehab Days	23,600	
Acute Rehab Admissions	1,500	
Acute Rehab Average LOS	16.1	days
Total Acute Days	339,700	
Total Acute Admissions	65,000	
Total Acute Average LOS	5.2	days
Subacute Days	106,800	
Subacute Admissions	9,000	
Subacute Average LOS	11.9	days
Home Health Visits	522,300	
Home Health Patients	17,000	
Home Health Visits/Patient	30.7	
Inpatient Surgery Cases	22,600	
Outpatient Surgery Cases	46,600	
Total Surgery Cases	69,200	
Physician Office Visits	2,054,200	
Emergency Room Visits	142,300	
Hospital Outpatient Clinic Visits	165,000	

☐ ABC Health System's marketshare, 1997

market performance to the future expected levels yields important findings about future competitive needs and provides a forward-looking perspective of the competitive fitness of the organization.

As the examples demonstrate, these analytic exercises are both highly future oriented and very dynamic from a competitive analysis standpoint. This type of modeling can greatly enhance the results of the competitive advantage and disadvantage analysis by injecting a healthy and appropriate dose of futurism.

RESOLUTION OF PLANNING ISSUES

The final task of the situation analysis is to determine what critical planning issues need resolution during the strategic planning process. All of the preceding analysis is input to this final result. The determination is a subjective one that usually evolves through an iterative process of some or all of the following steps, depending on the size and complexity of the organization, its issues, and the extent of participative process used in strategic planning. After the planning analyst or planning staff select an initial list of issues, senior management team members, individually or collectively, may then review and revise the list of issues. The list may then go back for the strategic planning committee members, individually or collectively, to do the same. The issue listing may then be accepted as a basis for moving forward or returned to the planning or senior management staff for further work.

The outputs from the situation analysis may be quite diverse. A framework for categorizing the types of critical planning issues that emerge is shown in Figure 3.4. Typical critical planning issues that are common to strategic plans of the late 1990s are:

- survival as an independent entity;
- competitive cost positioning;
- market penetration and managed care approach;
- teaching role; and
- building an effective multi-provider (integrated delivery) system.

Only a limited number of planning issues can and should be dealt with effectively in the strategic planning process. The temptation in the situation analysis is to enumerate dozens of "important" issues that need to be resolved to ensure future success, sacrificing strategic precision in the name of comprehensiveness and political expediency.

Table 3.1 ABC Health System Strategic Planning Indicators and Their Implications

Indicator	Current Level	Benchmark or Best Practice Standard	Expected or Target Level, 2000–2005	Strategic Implications and Responses
Acute inpatient admissions per 1000 population	Service Area 103 Region 117 State 125 United States 132	95	100–110	More complex inpatient case mix and higher percentage of 65+ admissions More complex outpatient cases
Acute inpatient days per 1000 population	Service Area 904 Region 880 State 823 United States 831	440	500–575	Significantly fewer acute inpatients beds Likelihood that several smaller hospitals will cease to provide acute inpatient care Increased demand for post-acute services
ED visits per 1000 population	Service Area 357 Region 405 State 391 United States 359	200	225–260	Fast-track system for nonurgent ED patients More geographically distributed, more accessible to primary care
Subacute (skilled nursing) days per 1000 population	Service Area NA Region NA State NA United States NA	220	130–180	Higher transfer rates to subacute care Increased demand for subacute beds Need to create capacity to meet growing demand and ensure systemwide access
Average PMPM HMO premiums commercial insurers	Service Area 145 Region 145 State 125 United States 144	105	125	Per capita expenditures for healthcare will decrease as premium declines are passed on to providers
Health insurance premium allocation by expense category	State HMOs Hospital 29% Physician 42% Pharmacy 8% Other 4% Payor 17%	California HMOs 30% 37% 9% 3% 21%	30% 40% 10% 4% 16%	Fewer dollars available for acute hospital care as managed care takes hold Reallocation of resources to nonacute services will be essential
Case-mix adjusted expenses per adjusted discharge	Region 3,403 State 3,767 United States 4,025 Hospital A 3,619 Hospital B 4,176	3,100	Hospital A $3,300 Hospital B $3,000 System $3,200	System must curtail or reverse growth in total expenses despite continued increase in adjusted discharges
Percent of gross revenue from outpatient services	Region 40% State 31% United States 33% Hospital A 24% Hospital B 29%	50%	Hospital A 37% Hospital B 45% System 40%	Fill gaps in continuum of care Expand capacity of ambulatory services Partner with nonhospital providers who will otherwise compete for larger share of healthcare dollar

However, few healthcare organizations have so many strategic issues that they cannot be condensed to five to ten strategic issue categories at most. Failure to produce a limited number of issues to address

Figure 3.4   Results of Situation Analysis: Framework for Critical Issues Facing Healthcare Organizations

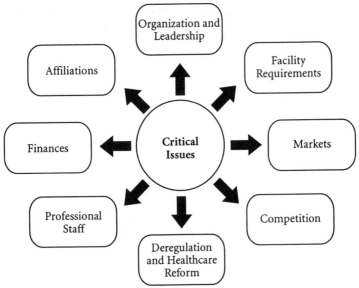

in subsequent planning activities almost always dooms the strategic planning process. It is impossible to address effectively an excessive number of issues concurrently and may confuse organization leadership about what issues are truly critical to strategic development.

A brief and high-level listing of planning issues requiring resolution is an excellent springboard to the next two planning activities: establishing overall or corporate strategic direction and formulating core strategies. A short list of key planning issues reduces voluminous data and information collected during the situation analysis to a manageable amount and energizes the organization leadership to move forward on strategic planning with a clear focus on issues of immense value to the organization.

Suggested Readings

Amara, R. 1988. "Health Care Tomorrow." *The Futurist* (November/December): 16–20.

Coile, R. 1986. *The New Hospital: Future Strategies for a Changing Industry*. Rockville, MD: Aspen Publishers, Inc.

Goldsmith, J. 1989. "A Radical Prescription for Hospitals." *Harvard Business Review* 89 (3): 104–11.

Hamel, G., and C. K. Prahalad. 1994. "Competing for the Future." *Harvard Business Review* 72 (4): 122–28.

Hancock, T., and C. Bezold. 1994. "Possible Futures, Preferable Futures." *Healthcare Forum Journal* 37 (2): 23–29.

Klay, W. E. 1988. "Strategic Management and Futures Research." *Futures Research Quarterly* (Summer): 49–60.

Schnaars, S. P. 1989. *Megamistakes.* New York: The Free Press.

Schwartz, P. 1991. *The Art of the Long View.* New York: Doubleday Currency.

Valins, M. S., and D. Salter. 1996. *Futurecare.* Cambridge, MA: Blackwell Science Ltd.

CHAPTER 4

Activity II: Identifying Strategic Direction

THE SECOND activity of the strategic planning process, identifying strategic direction, initiates in earnest the process of looking forward to frame what the organization's future might be. This activity sets high-level direction, encompassing mission, vision, values, and key overall organization strategies. Subsequent activities address important components of future direction and the particulars of implementation. Figure 4.1 provides a context for the principal outputs of the strategic plan included in this and subsequent chapters.

Much has been written in the strategic planning literature about the importance of a clear mission and vision to the organization's future success. Donaldson (1995) notes that to be effective, every organization needs a clear, unambiguous strategic mission statement and top management with the authority and ability to carry it out.[1] Campbell (1993) refers to organization vision as the foundation of the planning process that drives the development of broad strategies for attaining measurable organizational goals.[2] Coile (1994) describes the importance of vision using an analogy, stating that the interrelationship between vision and strategy is an arrow-to-target process. A shared vision is the target, while strategic planning is the arrow.[3] There are, however, caveats to developing mission and vision statements. Allen and Benson (1995) emphasize that the vision must be emotionally inspiring and personally fulfilling,[4] but according to Kaplan and Norton (1996), many vision statements are too lofty and fail to translate easily into operational terms that provide guides for action.[5] Beckham (1991) indicates that many mission statements are not relevant and lack a sense of direction or differentiation.[6]

Most often, healthcare organizations that clearly express their basic purpose in a mission statement, and have a good picture of what they want their organization to look like in five to ten years in a vision statement, stand a better chance of being able to articulate and implement the more specific components of the strategic plan, and realize the vision they have articulated. Failure to specify a mission that is compelling and unique to the healthcare organization, or define a vision that is clear and exciting, renders attempts to resolve strategic issues and make progress toward a better future extremely difficult.

ASSUMPTIONS ABOUT THE FUTURE

Market forecasts and planning issues are the two important products of the Activity I situation analysis, which allow the environmental context to be set for discussion and determination of mission and vision. The market forecasts present alternative views of broad environmental conditions that will affect organization behavior and performance in the future. The planning issues highlight aspects of future environmental conditions and organization characteristics that are of particular concern in setting organization direction.

Much planning by healthcare organizations and the general business community in the past has been predicated on one view of the future environment, usually linear extrapolations of the past, rather than evaluating a wide range of possible futures. The upheavals in healthcare and other industries illustrate how this singular view of the future has led to major errors in organization strategy and legitimate concern about the wisdom of planning for the future within a limited environmental context. General Motors failed in the 1970s to explore fully the impact of OPEC (Organization of Petroleum Exporting Countries), globalization, environmentalism, and the importance of quality and speed in manufacturing.[7] In the 1980s, IBM and Digital Equipment Corporation failed to account for the consequences of personal computers.[8] According to Hamel and Prahalad (1994), "If senior executives don't have reasonably detailed answers to the 'future' questions, and if the answers they have are not significantly different from the 'today' answers, there is little chance that their companies will remain market leaders."[9]

Planning for the future within a narrow, limited environmental context may have been acceptable in the more static, highly regulated healthcare environment prevalent through the early 1990s and

Figure 4.1 Planning Terminology and Definitions

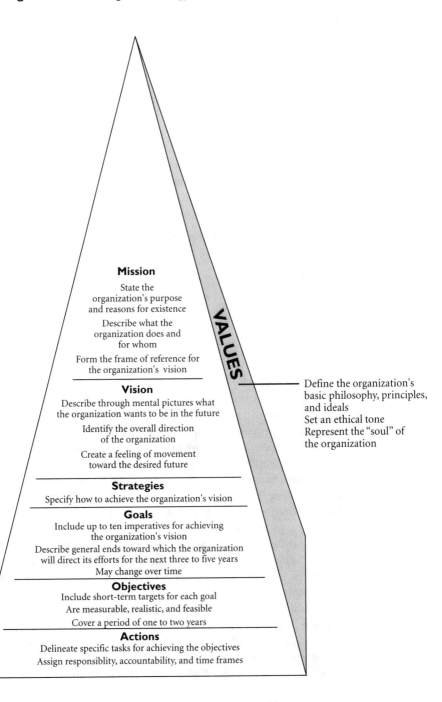

Mission

State the organization's purpose and reasons for existence

Describe what the organization does and for whom

Form the frame of reference for the organization's vision

Vision

Describe through mental pictures what the organization wants to be in the future

Identify the overall direction of the organization

Create a feeling of movement toward the desired future

Strategies

Specify how to achieve the organization's vision

Goals

Include up to ten imperatives for achieving the organization's vision

Describe general ends toward which the organization will direct its efforts for the next three to five years

May change over time

Objectives

Include short-term targets for each goal

Are measurable, realistic, and feasible

Cover a period of one to two years

Actions

Delineate specific tasks for achieving the objectives

Assign responsiblity, accountability, and time frames

VALUES

Define the organization's basic philosophy, principles, and ideals

Set an ethical tone

Represent the "soul" of the organization

beyond, in some of the most highly regulated states. However, it is no longer sensible and constitutes one of the main differences between contemporary strategic planning methods and those of the very recent past.

To ensure that a broader perspective is adopted, it is critical to define and discuss alternative futures in the fullest possible way before mission and vision can be appropriately determined. While this task could take place in Activity I, it is often better to approach it with a fresh perspective in Activity II, unencumbered by the accumulated data on the past, which limit the freer thinking required in this task. It may even be necessary to revise or fine-tune some of the products of the situation analysis after completing this task.

An excellent reference to draw on in developing alternative future scenarios is Peter Schwartz's *The Art of the Long View*.[10] Schwartz recommends the following steps in scenario development:

1. Identify the focal issue or decision.
2. Select a key focus in the local environment.
3. Determine the driving forces.
4. Rank by importance and uncertainty.
5. Select scenario logics.
6. Flesh out the scenarios.
7. Derive implications.
8. Select leading indicators and signposts.

This approach enables diverse alternative futures to be considered and seriously analyzed by organization leadership with a composite scenario distilled from this broad view of the future. In contrast, the typical approach used by most healthcare organizations today explicitly or implicitly relies on the planning staff to develop a single future environmental scenario by extrapolating current trends and incorporating "hot" issues of the present. For example, the proposed Clinton healthcare reform legislation was the centerpiece of most healthcare providers' future scenarios in 1993.

Regardless of which approach is used in this task, the result should be an explicit set of underlying assumptions about the future upon which the mission and vision will be based. Figure 4.2 presents an example of the nature and degree of detail of the assumptions that are useful as a precursor to the mission and vision determination process. As the example illustrates, the assumptions should be stated quite briefly to avoid unnecessarily complicating the perspective of the future environment in which the organization will operate. This concise, simple summary of a potential future environment is a

Figure 4.2 Example Assumptions about the Future Market: Year 2000

Major assumptions about the western North Carolina market in the year 2000 were developed to provide a framework for strategy:
• HMO* penetration in western North Carolina will approach 50 percent; on balance, care will be moderately managed.
• Systems will compete on both cost and quality parameters.
• Physicians will organize for practice and contracting purposes.
• Specialist utilization will decrease, significantly reducing physician incomes.
• The shift toward nonacute care will accelerate.

---

*HMO–health maintenance organization.
Source: Mission–St. Joseph's Health System, 1996.

powerful guide for consideration or, in many cases, reconsideration of organization mission and vision.

DEVELOPMENT OF THE MISSION STATEMENT

Most healthcare organizations have an existing statement of mission. In these cases, the starting point for the mission determination task needs to be the current statement. There are two main problems with most mission statements developed by healthcare organizations in recent years. First, they are often too lengthy and cumbersome, and second, the mission is often confused with strategy.

Effective mission statements are brief and fundamental statements of organization purpose that conform to the guidelines listed in Figure 4.1. A mission statement should clearly communicate to the board, employees, and other internal and external constituencies why the organization exists and what important purpose it intends to achieve. To accomplish this task, the mission statement must be brief and to the point. Many experts believe that the most effective mission statements are, at most, one sentence in length. Several examples of recently developed mission statements for healthcare organizations are presented in Figure 4.3.

Development of the mission statement can occur in many ways, but most organizations include significant input from the board since this is the board's most fundamental contribution to organization policy and strategic direction. Two to three sessions with the strategic planning committee, which are at least partly devoted to a discussion of mission, are usually sufficient to gain the input required to draft or redraft a statement that will be embraced by the board as the cornerstone of the strategic plan. These sessions ordinarily encompass:

- scenario development and generation of a composite future scenario;

- review of the definition of a mission statement and examination of the current statement;

- review of other healthcare organizations' mission statements; and

- review and modification of a new draft mission statement.

One note of caution is needed regarding the mission statement. It is not productive for the strategic planning committee or board to "wordsmith" the proposed mission statement. These groups should concentrate on what the mission statement is trying to convey, with discussion focusing on substantive changes in content. It is cumbersome, tedious, and ultimately unproductive for a strategic planning committee or board to rewrite, in whole or in part, the mission statement in a group discussion. Drafting or redrafting this document should be left to an individual or small group.

Figure 4.3 Mission Statements

KidsPeace
Give kids confidence to overcome crisis.
Source: KidsPeace, 1996.

St. David's Health Care System
St. David's Health Care System is a community-owned resource which strives to meet the health care needs of the Austin area through the provision of health services, leadership, and collaboration.
Source: St. David's Health Care System, 1992.

Mission–St. Joseph's Health System
We bring together the people, the caring cultures, and the values of our founding hospitals and join with others in meeting the health needs of our community and the region. We make health care measurably more accessible and affordable, continually improve the quality of our services, and promote wellness and the roles of both the individual and the community in achieving improved health.
Source: Mission–St. Joseph's Health System, 1996.

DEVELOPMENT OF THE
VISION STATEMENT ············

The task of developing a vision statement is usually carried out concurrently with the development of the mission statement and follows the same process and general principles. Many organizations also have existing statements of future vision, but where the mission statement is not time-limited, vision statements refer to a particular future point or period in time and generally must be updated and revised with each full strategic planning process. Unlike the mission statement, the current vision statement will probably require substantial change if it is to be an effective guide for the organization's future direction. And, similar to the mission statement, many current statements of organization vision share the two main problems that recent mission statements have—cumbersome length and inappropriate inclusion of strategy.

Effective vision statements conform to the guidelines listed in Figure 4.1, and are often brief, single-sentence statements of desired high-level organization characteristics at a distant point in the future, usually ten years. The vision statement should be a vehicle to communicate to internal constituencies a preferred, future state of the organization. It should be a challenge given current circumstances and conditions, and it should represent such an exciting and desirable state of being that it motivates and energizes all elements of the organization to reach it through the more detailed strategies and actions that follow. Several examples of healthcare organization vision statements that conform to this description are presented in Figure 4.4. The process comments related to the mission statement apply in this task, too. Interactions between the board, strategic planning committee, and other key leaders should produce and refine an effective vision statement, without excessive attention to "wordsmithing."

DEVELOPMENT OF OVERALL
ORGANIZATION STRATEGY ············

Both the mission and vision address the "what" of future strategic direction. However, many healthcare organizations cannot or do not distinguish between the "what" and "how" of future direction, and inappropriately include strategy in mission or vision statements. It is often difficult for organizations to distinguish a principal means (i.e., strategy) to accomplish the ends (i.e., mission and vision) they have articulated. Typically, multiple and diverse overall strategies may be set forth, the result of which is really no strategy at all. Thus, overall organization strategy is often the least clearly defined element of future strategic direction.

Miles and Snow (1978) developed a typology that measures a hospital's strategic orientation, which includes prospectors, defenders, analyzers, and reactors. A *prospector* is defined as an organization that makes frequent changes in and additions to its services and markets, and consistently responds rapidly to market opportunities by being the first to provide a new service or develop a new market. A *defender* offers a fairly stable set of services to defined markets and tends to ignore changes that do not directly affect current operations, focusing instead on doing its best in the current arena. An *analyzer* also maintains a relatively stable base of services, but selectively develops new services or markets, like the prospector. However, the analyzer rarely is the first to provide new services or expand into new markets, choosing instead to monitor actions of others, and following with a more well-thought-through approach. A *reactor* is an organization that does not appear to respond consistently to changes in the market and seems to lack a coherent strategy. The reactor may, on occasion, be an early entrant into a new market or service, but usually is forced into action by external events or after considerable evidence of potential for success.[11]

It may be difficult for a healthcare organization to articulate its strategy as other than prospector, and as Shortell, Morrison, and Friedman (1990) point out, since few healthcare organizations are really following a prospector strategy, this may explain part of the confusion about overall strategy that healthcare providers evidence.[12]

Another framework for overall strategy that is prevalent in general business, developed by Porter, suggests that companies must

Figure 4.4 Vision Statements

KidsPeace
To turn a generation of kids in crisis into a nation of kids who overcome.
Source: KidsPeace, 1996.

St. David's Health Care System
St. David's envisions an integrated health care delivery system that provides select specialty services in a high-quality and cost-effective manner.
Source: St. David's Health Care System, 1992.

Mission–St. Joseph's Health System
We will be a leader and innovator in linking a full range of health care providers and services that is uniquely responsive to the people and cultures we serve. We will distinguish ourselves by achieving improved health in our community and the region.
Source: Mission–St. Joseph's Health System, 1996.

---

follow three principal strategies (singly or in combination) to create a defendable position: overall cost leadership, differentiation, and focus.[13] The *overall cost leadership* strategy is achieved through a set of aggressive policies that ensure construction of efficient facilities, pursue rigorous cost reductions, and control costs and overhead. *Differentiation* of a product or service offering means creating something that is perceived industrywide as being unique. The differentiation strategy does not ignore costs, but they are not the primary strategic focus. The third strategy is to *focus* on a particular buyer or geographic market. While the low-cost and differentiation strategies try to achieve objectives industrywide, the focus strategy aims to serve a particular target well, and policies are developed with this in mind. The premise is that the organization is then able to serve its narrow target focus more effectively than those competing broadly.

Regardless of which strategy framework is adopted by the organization, a clear choice must be made from among available alternative future strategies if the organization is to have a high probability of realizing its vision. A principal strategy needs to be selected and articulated to all affected internal organization constituencies as part of the strategic direction.

The process of developing overall organization strategy can be quite similar to that described previously for the mission and vision statements. The main difference is in the degree to which this statement emanates from planning staff and top management versus the strategic planning committee and the board.

As the organization moves more into the "how" of strategic planning, the roles and responsibility of management will expand. The strategic planning committee and the board may have significant input to the overall strategy statement because it is a major policy statement on a par with the mission and vision, but it is at this point the transition from board-driven strategic planning to staff-driven strategic planning begins to take place.

DEVELOPMENT OF THE VALUES STATEMENT

As Figure 4.1 illustrates, the values statement is the underpinning of the entire strategic direction and plan. Like the mission and vision statements, many organizations have already developed a statement of values. In the absence of significant organization or environmental changes, this statement is relatively timeless and may not require major modification.

With the increasing number of mergers, other forms of affiliation, and emergence of integrated delivery systems, few healthcare organizations will be untouched by the waves of change now sweeping the industry. In these new arrangements, diverse organization cultures are brought together, and existing values are blended, or in some cases imposed, on the new entity. The issue of the character of the organization culture that is desirable in the new entity and how this is represented to employees and other important stakeholders is at the core of what the values statement represents.

In stable, successful healthcare organizations, a values statement can probably best be gleaned from organization behavior. Observance of the day-to-day practices of the employees and of board policy and performance will lead to a fairly clear picture of the values of the organization. This values statement can be fine-tuned by leadership to reflect some minor modification of organization behavior and then serve as the product for this task.

For other healthcare organizations, a values statement will probably need to be developed through a top-down process, similar to that recommended for the mission statement. Where new or significantly different organization values are necessary, leadership must determine what the current organization values are (which may differ across recently combined entities) and how they have come into being. Then the organization must conduct a self-examination to create a new values statement for the future. An example of a recently developed values statement typical of what many healthcare organizations aspire to is illustrated in Figure 4.5.

MOVING TO THE NEXT ACTIVITY

Four critical outputs—mission, vision, strategy, and values statements—compose the statement of strategic direction for the organization and are produced during Activity II of the strategic planning

Figure 4.5 Values Statement

Concern . . . for the total well-being of people in our community and our corporate family.

Professionalism . . . in dealing with the public and each other.

Respect . . . for individual dignity and for the needs and gifts of all with whom we come in contact.

Charity . . . toward others and from others.

Collaboration . . . with and through our employees and affiliated physicians.

Satisfaction . . . from serving others, and the way others view our service to them.

Source: Pinnacle Health System, 1996.

process. With the description of strategic direction completed, it is possible to move productively into the next level of detail of strategic planning—the goals and strategies to address the remaining important issues defined in Activity I.

Notes

1. Donaldson, G. 1995. "A New Tool for Boards: The Strategic Audit." *Harvard Business Review* 73 (4): 100.
2. Campbell, A. B. 1993. "Strategic Planning in Health Care: Methods and Applications." *Quality Management in Health Care* 1 (4): 14.
3. Coile, R. C., Jr. 1994. "Making Strategic Planning a Vision-Driven Process." *Hospital Strategy Report* 6 (10): 8.
4. Allen, D., and J. Benson. 1995. "New Year's Brings New Roles and Responsibilities." *Health Care Strategic Management* 13 (1): 7.
5. Kaplan, R. S., and D. P. Norton. 1996. "Using the Balanced Scorecard as a Strategic Management System." *Harvard Business Review* 74 (1): 76.
6. Beckham, J. D. 1991. "Strategic Thinking and the Road to Relevance." *Healthcare Forum* 34 (6): 38.
7. Schoemaker, P. J. H. 1995. "Scenario Planning: A Tool for Strategic Thinking." *Sloan Management Review* 36 (2): 25.
8. Ibid.
9. Hamel, G., and C. K. Prahalad. 1994. "Competing for the Future." *Harvard Business Review* 72 (4): 127.
10. Schwartz, P. 1991. *The Art of the Long View*. New York: Doubleday Currency.
11. Miles, R. E., and C. C. Snow. 1978. *Organizational Strategy, Structure, and Process*. New York: McGraw-Hill.
12. Shortell, S. M., E. M. Morrison, and B. Friedman. 1990. *Strategic Choices for America's Hospitals*. San Francisco: Jossey-Bass Publishers.
13. Porter, M. E. 1980. *Competitive Strategy*. New York: The Free Press.

CHAPTER 5

Activity III: Developing Core Business Strategies

FROM VISION TO GOALS

WITH OVERALL organization direction defined, goals and objectives for the organization and its future strategic development can be determined. It should be clear from the preceding chapter that to achieve the vision of the next five to ten years, significant progress must be made in a number of key areas. These subareas of overall strategy are derived from the strategic issues determined in Activity I.

For many organizations, the most difficult part of strategic planning is moving from the vision to the next level of detail: the goals. The temptation is to identify literally hundreds of areas in which critical activity needs to occur to achieve the vision. The result is an unwieldy and ultimately unimplementable plan. Strategic planning at its essence is the process of making difficult choices among competing priorities and focusing the organization's limited resources in those areas with the greatest payoff. If strategic planning is to be effective, that focus needs to be maintained throughout the process, but especially in this transition from vision to goals. A successful organization generally is able to identify no more than ten and, preferably, as few as five goals that are priorities for realizing the vision.

Moving from vision to goals is most readily accomplished in a three-phase process:

- determination of strategic issues;
- white papers on strategic issues; and
- identification of goals.

Determination of Strategic Issues

Strategic issues embody those areas in which action is probably needed to realize the vision. Strategic issues are determined by examining the mission, vision, and key organization strategy in light of the planning issues defined in the situation analysis. Often, the planning issues themselves constitute the strategic issues for the organization, but they may need to be reshaped because of conclusions reached in the strategic direction phase of the planning process. In any event, reviewing the planning issues is a good starting place for determining the organization's strategic issues.

Planning staff or a small group of senior management should narrow the number of potential strategic issues down to no more than ten and present the findings of their analyses to the strategic planning committee for review and modification. It is important to specify why the selected areas are strategically important, and why other areas are not. An example of a representative list of strategic issues that resulted from such a process is shown in Figure 5.1.

White Papers on Strategic Issues

Once the strategic issues are agreed upon, there are a number of potential paths to move from issues to goals. A more process-intensive approach, rather than a less process-intensive one, is more likely to identify the best goals (and the best objectives and actions) and to build support for plan implementation and action. Preparing white papers, or in-depth reports, on strategic issues is an option to help distinguish and prioritize alternatives.

Clearly, the most process-intensive approach will require more time to complete, typically as long as three to four months. The least process-intensive approach can be completed in as little as a month

Figure 5.1   Strategic Issues

St. David's Health Care System

- Integration
- Charitable mission
- Inpatient services
- Ambulatory care
- Centers of excellence
- Value
- Financial viability

Source: St. David's Health Care System, 1992.

or less. If the time frame for planning is a concern, the approach selected for this activity should be carefully considered.

There are three basic paths (with a number of variations) that can be followed.

1. **Move directly from strategic issues to goals.** Planning staff, senior management, or the strategic planning committee deduce the goals without further analysis or process.

2. **Prepare white papers on strategic issues.** Planning staff prepares position papers on each strategic issue, and recommends goals for review and modification by senior management and the strategic planning committee.

3. **Convene task forces to prepare white papers.** Similar to the above, except that a multifaceted group of organization representatives is convened for a limited period of time to assist in preparing the white papers.

The third alternative has an additional benefit in that it exposes important organization stakeholders to the outline of the strategic plan that is likely to result from the planning process, and constructively engages them in further definition of organization strategy in areas of both significance and relevance to them personally. If this is the path chosen, a few guidelines about how to proceed are in order.

Assemble the task forces with care.

Unfortunately, there is no fool-proof formula for assembling task forces, but recognizing what objectives your organization is trying to accomplish and the potential incompatibility of all the objectives is a good starting point. A number of sometimes conflicting objectives may be accomplished in selecting task force members. Those objectives might include:

- gaining broad representation from potentially affected constituencies;
- having enough diversity so that the task force is not biased toward any single perspective;
- achieving relatively good personal chemistry among the members;
- assembling a task force not too large as to be unwieldy (there are few task forces that are too small);
- selecting members who are interested enough to participate actively; and
- choosing a leader who will lead, but not dominate.

The task forces typically will meet three to four times over a six- to eight-week period. The members should understand and appreciate that their charge is time-limited, and that they are not making decisions, only presenting alternatives and making recommendations to the strategic planning committee.

Provide guidelines and support to task forces.

First, although active participation and free-flowing discussion are to be encouraged, some structure and staff support are necessary to achieve sound outputs and leave the participants feeling that they were constructively involved in the process. Expectations for the task forces need to be defined clearly at the outset, including time frame for deliberation, questions to answer or issues to address, and likely structure of the output needed. Figures 5.2 and 5.3 exhibit samples of information that might be provided to task forces. Data and other relevant information collected in earlier activities of the planning process should be assembled and provided to task force members in advance of their first meeting. The planning staff should be identified as staff support to the task forces and play a major role in logistical support, data support, and production of the white papers themselves.

Identification of Goals

Ideally, each white paper will thoroughly review all aspects of the strategic issue and present recommendations that allow a goal, or occasionally multiple goals, to be readily identified. It is the strategic planning committee's job, with appropriate planning staff and management support, to select a goal that will constructively and creatively deal with the strategic issue (and assist in achieving some part of the vision or at least make significant strides in that direction). Typically, each task force leader will present his or her team's report to the strategic planning committee for review, modification, and ultimate acceptance. At that time, or in a subsequent meeting, a potential goal will be identified, discussed, and modified before approval by the strategic planning committee. Figure 5.4 presents goals that were defined for the strategic issues listed in Figure 5.1. The completion of this task is significant in that it puts in place the final piece of the strategic plan with which the board should be concerned.

Collectively, the mission, vision, values, strategy, and goals constitute the "policy" portion of the plan, while the remaining components, objectives and actions, are tactical and operational in nature. It may be helpful to think about the strategic plan as composed of two parts: strategy, which has been the subject of chapters 4 and 5 until this point, and the management action plan, which remains to be completed.

Figure 5.2 Task Force Overview

Strategic Issue	Issues to Be Explored	Proposed Leadership and Membership Profile
1. Primary care network	• Size and distribution of the network • Operational and financial expectations • Mechanisms for incorporating physicians into the network	Leader: Primary care physician Members: Primary care physicians Managed care marketing staff Senior Pinnacle management Practice managers
2. Cost management	• Cost target required to compete successfully • Schedule to attain targeted costs • Approaches to cost management and reduction	Leader: Chief financial officer (CFO) Members: Department chairs Senior Pinnacle management
3. Medical education	• Role of medical education within Pinnacle • Expectations of medical education and criteria for evaluating residencies • Need for an academic affiliation	Leader: Teaching physician Members: Physicians trained at Pinnacle programs Other physicians Senior Pinnacle management

Source: Pinnacle Health System, 1996.

Unfortunately, few not-for-profit boards understand or appreciate this distinction. Although the work of the strategic planning committee as a whole should be wrapped up at this point, and management should take responsibility for completing the remaining plan tasks and components, most strategic planning committees continue to function in an increasingly dysfunctional way until the plan is entirely complete. A compromise may be in order here. Rather than finish the committee's work at this point, or allow it to continue to provide oversight in a manner similar to that done in prior tasks, thank the committee for completing the overwhelming majority of its important work and offer to reconvene it when the objectives and actions are drafted. At that point, management can present its draft management action plan and an executive summary of the plan to

Figure 5.3 White Paper Outline

Issue I: Name

- Issue definition
- Background (including importance of resolving the issue)
- Analysis of issue components and alternative approaches
- Findings and observations
- Recommendations
- Implementation considerations

---

the committee. Following review by the committee, the action plan and executive summary are submitted to the full board for approval and adoption.

OBJECTIVES AND ACTIONS: THE MANAGEMENT ACTION PLAN

If the approach suggested above is followed, the remaining planning tasks are carried out under the direction of senior management.

Figure 5.4 Goals

Integration
  A comprehensive system of integrated services and settings capable of providing health care for a population of at least 250,000

Charitable Mission
  Advancement of community health status through investment in health education, health promotion, and charity care

Inpatient Services
  Stable or increasing marketshares in major inpatient services

Ambulatory Care
  Ambulatory care leadership, doubling outpatient revenues by 1997

Centers of Excellence
  Neuro/Ortho/Rehab/Psych center of distinction that captures one-third of the neurosciences market in central Texas

Value
  Highest health care value as measured by favorable cost per case and high customer satisfaction

Financial Viability
  Financial viability in terms of an annual return on equity of 10 percent and return on net revenues of 3 percent

---

Source: St. David's Health Care System, 1992.

These tasks typically involve broader representation of management team members than has been the case up to this point.

Essentially, each goal needs to be dissected into smaller more manageable components:

- objectives, which represent short-term targets in each goal area; and

- actions, which are the principal activities that need to be accomplished to achieve the objectives.

The objectives and actions collectively compose the near-term "game plan" to move the organization's strategic plan forward.

As with other critical strategic planning tasks, a choice must be made about the nature and extent of desirable participation. Developing appropriate, productive objectives and actions requires that the people charged with carrying out the management action plan be involved in creating it. Clearly, it is possible, and in some situations it may even be desirable, to create a management action plan without much process or participation, but these situations should be the exception rather than the rule.

Some or all of the following steps might be followed to develop objectives and actions:

- designate a member of the senior management group to oversee preparation of objectives and actions for each goal, based on his or her areas of responsibility and interest;

- create a management task force, or consult individuals for each goal area to assist in developing objectives and actions for each goal;

- convene a meeting of senior management one to three times during this process to review progress, critique each other's work, identify areas of overlap in the action plans, and make necessary adjustments;

- estimate resource requirements, identify the person(s) or group(s) responsible for overseeing implementation, and determine time frames for implementation once objectives and draft actions are designed; and

- prepare a completed management action plan as the collective work product of each individual senior manager's efforts (compiled as a companion document to the policy and strategic planning output).

An example of objectives and actions for a given goal is presented in Figure 5.5.

One final issue in completing this activity is deserving of some discussion. There is great controversy among strategic planners about

Figure 5.5 Management Action Plan Output

Goal 4: Ambulatory Care Leadership, Doubling Outpatient Revenues by 1997*

4.1 Develop an integrated ambulatory care system representative of campuswide services

    4.1.1 Establish a task force to address ambulatory needs, barriers, and opportunities

        4.1.1.1 Identify organization and leadership

    4.1.2 Complete an ambulatory care strategic and business plan

        4.1.2.1 Coordinate acute care with rehabilitation and psychiatry components

        4.1.2.2 Resolve product-line or system orientation (see 1.4.1)

        4.1.2.3 Provide information system specifications to management information system long-range plan (See 7.2.1)

    4.1.3 Identify site(s) for potential on-campus outpatient center and network (see 1.1.6)

    4.1.4 Evaluate and implement workers' compensation program (see 3.2.2.3)

    4.1.5 Resolve oncology program issues (i.e., collaborate or compete)

    4.1.6 Market systemwide ambulatory capabilities (see 4.2.6)

4.2 Sponsor outpatient presence through metropolitan statistical area

    4.2.1 Complete off-campus portion of ambulatory care strategic plan

        4.2.1.1 Resolve product-line or system orientation

    4.2.2 Support off-campus physicians

        4.2.2.1 Determine and establish physician needs and interests (see 6.3.1.3)

        4.2.2.2 Implement physician development plan (see 1.1.2)

    4.2.3 Expand home care program

    4.2.4 Expand psychiatry outpatient continuum

        4.2.4.1 Evaluate feasibility of group home, residential, or in-home programs

        4.2.4.2 Develop implementation program

    4.2.5 Expand rehabilitation outpatient continuum

        4.2.5.1 Evaluate feasibility of group home, resident, or in-home programs

        4.2.5.2 Identify location for potential comprehensive outpatient rehabilitation facility

        4.2.5.3 Develop implementation program

    4.2.6 Market systemwide ambulatory capabilities (see 4.2.1)

Source: St. David's Health Care System, 1992.

*References to additional objectives and actions have been left intact, although only objectives and actions from this section are reprinted here.

the depth and breadth of financial analysis that is appropriate in the strategic planning process. Clearly, a minimalist approach is recommended in this book, while others believe something close to a financial feasibility forecast is necessary. Current thinking on this subject, as embodied in much of the literature referenced in

Chapter 1, is consistent with the approach recommended here. The strategic plan should have a high-level strategy focus. Any substantial financial analysis should occur in implementation. However, one note of caution is important. The approach recommended in this book is one that is continually vigilant and cognizant of the need to recognize resource limitations, make choices, and focus effort. This can be accomplished with a process that has financial awareness and concerns as part of its infrastructure so that financial implications are implicitly part of each step of the process. If this degree of financial awareness and astuteness is not routinely part of the organization's work, some substantive financial tasks may need to be included in the strategic planning process.

CHAPTER 6

Activity IV: Transitioning to Implementation

IMPLEMENTATION FRAMEWORK

THE LAST substantive strategic plan task is the preparation of an implementation framework. This task involves taking the actions identified as the final output in the previous chapter and putting them into a framework that facilitates implementation and ongoing monitoring of implementation progress. At a minimum, each action should be assigned to a primary party who will be responsible for directing and scheduling implementation. Some implementation frameworks may include additional information such as secondary parties or groups that will support implementation; incremental operational or capital resource requirements and time frames; approval requirements; significant decision-making needs; timing; and so forth. A basic implementation framework is illustrated in Figure 6.1.

With implementation nearing, the typical strategic planning process will involve additional members of the healthcare organization's management team. As noted earlier, during the course of the strategic plan development process primary responsibility shifts from the board, whose focus is on the early strategic policy recommendations, to the senior management, whose responsibility it will be to implement these policies and provide consistent strategic direction to all the operational entities of the organization, and finally to a broad group of middle management and staff who will act as the front-line implementation team. If implementation is to be effective, these implementation team members need to understand the aspects of the strategic plan that have been developed largely by the board and senior management, and they need to actively participate in shaping those parts of the plan that they will be principally responsible for (i.e., actions and schedule). At this point in the process, broad-based involvement of middle managers and others is not only appropriate but critical.

Often, a senior manager will be assigned primary responsibility for implementation activity related to a specific goal and will assemble an implementation team to work on the goal. Depending on the complexity of the assigned area and scope of implementation activities required, the team may consist of as few as 2 to 3 individuals or as many as 20. During this final task of the strategic plan development process, each implementation team ordinarily will meet two to three times to flesh out the initial implementation framework. Every organization operates in its own unique manner. Some work

Figure 6.1   Strategic Plan Implemention Outline

Objective I: Design system infrastructure, particularly information systems	
Action	**Completion Time**
1. Prepare a plan for developing the patient care management system	4/97–9/97
a. Requirements defined	
b. Potential vendors identified	
c. Budget parameters identified	
d. Site visits and demonstrations	
e. Selection	
2. Ensure management and capital resources are committed to all components of the system as well as to system development	4/97–9/97
a. Time commitment identified	
b. Team leaders established	
c. Target cost estimated	
d. Impact on financial plan and budget analyzed	
3. Define the mechanisms for measuring the health status of area residents	9/97–12/97
a. Research models	
b. Solicit input from MAHEC and other Health Partners resources	
c. Develop measurement method	
d. Establish frequency	
e. Secure ongoing funding	

Source: Mission–St. Joseph's Health System, 1996.

best with loose frameworks, similar to Figure 6.1, while others may significantly expand this chart with additional implementation detail for each action. However the organization decides it is best to proceed, the goal must not be lost in the process. Implementation should begin as rapidly as possible, often before the plan is actually adopted by the organization, and should proceed as envisioned, with modifications as necessary and appropriate, so that the organization's strategic direction is accomplished.

ADOPTION OF THE
STRATEGIC PLAN · · · · · · · · · · · ·

If planning activities have proceeded smoothly up until this point, adoption of the strategic plan is fairly simple and straightforward. The steps that need to be followed to formally approve the strategic plan include:

- preparation of an executive summary;
- preparation of the strategic plan document;
- resolution by the strategic planning committee recommending approval of the plan by the board;
- formal and informal educational sessions and presentations of the strategic plan to the board; and
- approval by the board of the strategic plan.

Preparation of an executive summary of the strategic plan is sometimes overlooked in the rush to move from planning to implementation. However, this document is often the only strategic plan output read by many board members and other important stakeholders. When new board members and senior staff members join the organization in the first few years following completion of the strategic plan, the executive summary of the strategic plan provides a critical perspective on both the organization and its strategic direction.

The executive summary should include the rationale for preparation of the strategic plan, background on the planning process used, major findings, and major recommendations. It is highly desirable for this executive summary to be no more than two to three pages in length. However, some organizations issue the executive summary as a stand-alone document with the strategic plan itself as a separate, companion document, which may be structured more as a white paper output from the strategic planning process, about five to ten pages long with perhaps a few brief appendixes.

Whether the executive summary is prepared as a stand-alone document or integrated into the strategic plan, a full strategic plan report should be prepared at the conclusion of the planning process.

The strategic plan report should include the outputs of all planning activities as well as a description of important process steps (e.g., interviews, retreats). This document serves as the record for all that occurred during the planning process and provides an excellent reference of analyses and supporting information that may be germane to implementation.

The complete strategic plan document usually is received in draft form by senior management and the strategic planning committee before being finalized. Most organizations provide a copy of the strategic plan report to all board members prior to discussion of approval of the plan by the board. The full report is also distributed to the senior management team. Further distribution of the report or the executive summary is discretionary depending on the sensitivity of material included in the report, extent of competition and potential for strategy "leaks," and the need-to-know of potential recipients of the plan itself.

Although it may only be a formality if the strategic planning process has proceeded smoothly, the procedure followed in nearly all healthcare organizations is for the strategic planning committee to formally recommend adoption of the plan to the board. As noted above, a draft document typically is received by the planning committee at its final committee meeting. Usually, limited changes in wording or format may be suggested by the committee, with the main purpose of the meeting to recommend the plan to the board for approval. Occasionally, this final meeting is also used to discuss next steps and implementation, and to outline how the committee will be involved in subsequent strategic plan updating or implementation monitoring.

In most healthcare organizations, at least one full presentation of the strategic plan to the board is provided prior to formal review by the board. This educational session, which may be conducted in a retreat format, provides an opportunity for the full board to review and question the plan's analyses, findings, and recommendations. This type of session is intended to increase the board's understanding of the plan and its implications for the organization and allow any important issues about the plan development process and subsequent implementation to surface and be discussed.

For most healthcare organizations, one educational session of this type is the only major activity required before formal board consideration of the plan. However, some organizations may require a second educational session, small group discussions, or one-to-one meetings between board members and the CEO. Senior management and leadership of the strategic planning committee must do whatever is necessary to ensure that board members understand

and support the strategic plan. Strategic planning leadership should be especially sensitive to board member's concerns, confusion, or discomfort and attempt to address directly board member's needs so that the full board is genuinely enthused about strategic plan adoption and implementation.

The board review and approval process of the strategic plan may encompass a limited number of steps carried out over a few weeks, or a significant number of steps over a few months. This is largely a function of the complexity of the plan, its recommendations, and organizational style, such as the degree of deliberateness in the review and approval process. Rarely are strategic plans not approved, although there are undoubtedly instances where the plan is rejected by the board at this point or returned to the planning staff or committee for major rework. If the staff and committee have done their jobs well, including gathering extensive input and communicating with all elements of organization leadership, the board approval process should proceed without any serious roadblocks.

Adoption of the strategic plan by the board should be a mere formality. If this is not the case at the time the strategic plan is brought forward for formal consideration, undoubtedly some of the preparation was lacking or sensitivity to board concerns was not appreciated.

UPDATING THE
STRATEGIC PLAN

In today's healthcare delivery environment, a comprehensive and thorough strategic planning process should result in a strategic plan that has a useful life of three to five years. Nonetheless, the plan will need to be updated or fine-tuned during that period. In fact, strategic planning should be viewed as an ongoing activity of the organization. Even in years when a full updating of the plan is not required, there should be an annual calendar of strategic planning activities, including limited update of the environmental assessment, modification of goals, and preparation of new or revised objectives and actions.

It is especially important to monitor progress in achieving strategic plan goals and objectives; in some cases, it may be necessary to abandon goals or objectives because they are not achievable or no longer desirable. As a result of implementation activities or strategic plan update analyses, secondary, contingency strategies or actions may need to be deployed, with the primary strategy or action de-emphasized or halted.

Two major planning-related activities should occur in the off-years when a comprehensive strategic planning process is not underway: updating and implementing the plan. In some organizations, responsibility for these activities is assigned to the same party, a group of senior management staff or the strategic planning committee. Even if the responsibilities for carrying out these activities are separated, the activities need to be linked and communication must occur regularly between the responsible parties.

In those years in which a limited update of the strategic plan occurs, it is still important to create a record of the update process and output (i.e., Strategic Plan Update for [year]) and, in some instances, to update the full board or formally modify the approved strategic plan. Many healthcare organizations now conduct an annual board retreat, which is a good forum for review of the year's progress and for setting direction for the next year.

CHAPTER 7

Special Process Considerations

RECENTLY AND in the foreseeable future, the planning process used during strategic planning is more important to the organization and the success of strategic planning than the strategic plan itself. Why is this the case? The increasing complexity of the healthcare environment and the growing vulnerability of healthcare organizations to environmental and competitive threats has made it far more challenging to come up with effective strategic plans. At the same time, the increasing size of healthcare organizations and the diversity and complexity of many of these organizations, especially the large multientity systems, has significantly increased communications difficulties and rendered these unwieldy organizations difficult to manage.

The planning process can be an important bridge to the many constituencies involved in these organizations and can facilitate better communication among staff as well as improved coherence in future operations. While the organization should certainly seek tangible outputs from strategic planning, the planning process presents important opportunities for improving communications across the organization, and forges new and stronger bonds among stakeholder individuals and groups to help ensure the organization's future viability.

With this in mind, this chapter addresses some of the critical elements of the planning process. While many of these elements have been mentioned in passing in previous chapters, the importance of a strong planning process calls for more extended discussion.

PLANNING RETREATS

Almost every strategic planning process will have at least one planning retreat. The retreat will usually bring together board members, physicians, and other clinicians and management in an extended planning session. Some retreats are intended for board members exclusively, others for members of different leadership groups. Depending on the organization's style and preferences, as well as the particular focus of the planning retreat, the retreat may be held off site and may even be carried out in a remote location and combined with social and recreational activities. Following is a review of the purposes of the different types of retreats that may be held during the strategic planning process.

Kickoff retreat

Some organizations use a retreat at the beginning of strategic planning to jump start the process and create enthusiasm and momentum. The agenda for this type of retreat may include some or all of the following:

- review of previous planning efforts, successes, and failures;
- review of the organization's recent performance;
- discussion of the organization's SWOTs; and
- identification on a preliminary basis of major planning issues.

Often, one or more outside keynote speakers will be used to discuss critical issues or challenges facing the organization. This type of retreat is a good vehicle for underscoring the importance of strategic planning and creating heightened interest in the planning process from the outset.

Midprocess retreat

At any number of points in the middle of the strategic planning process, retreats can be held to:

- focus on a particular issue of concern;
- have extended discussion that is not possible within a regular planning committee session;
- obtain broad-based input, including the planning committee as well as other important leaders not represented on the committee; or
- brainstorm about approaches to issues facing the organization.

External speakers may be used in midprocess retreats in a manner similar to kickoff retreats. The purpose of the midprocess retreat is information sharing, and it is rarely used for decision making or communicating "answers" to strategic planning issues at this stage in the process.

Concluding retreat

At or near the end of the strategic planning process, a retreat may be held to:

- obtain additional, broad-based input before finalizing the recommendations;
- communicate the answers (i.e., what the plan's key recommendations are);
- serve as a bridge to implementation, including strategizing about implementation opportunities and barriers; and
- build a broader consensus on the plan and its recommendations than that represented within the planning committee alone.

Often, this type of retreat will be developed to expose all members of the board to the strategic plan before it is brought to this group for formal consideration of its adoption. This type of retreat may also be used to signal the organization that planning is (temporarily) over, and implementation is about to begin.

As noted in earlier chapters, retreats may be held in off-years, when a full strategic planning effort is not undertaken, to accomplish any of the purposes cited above and to keep the planning process going even as the organization's efforts are primarily devoted to implementation.

RESEARCH APPROACHES

Much of the success of the strategic planning process is dependent on information gathering and involvement of key constituencies, which comes through various research efforts. The importance of constructive involvement of key constituencies in the strategic planning process cannot be overstated; implementation is dependent on a broad base of support for the plan's recommendations and actions. This support is only likely to occur if stakeholders believe they had a true opportunity to shape the results. A brief review of the range of research approaches used in strategic planning follows.

Interviews

Interviewing is typically part of every strategic planning process. Individual or group interviews usually occur early in the strategic planning process to gather information and demonstrate sensitivity to the perspectives of internal parties, but also to accomplish one or both of these purposes with external parties. Occasionally, interviews may be carried out during the middle of the process to gather additional information on issues of concern or involve select parties in review of alternative approaches for addressing particular issues.

Surveys

Surveys are the second most frequently employed technique, and are often used for information gathering early in the strategic planning process. Surveys may be carried out internally to gather broader input in a less expensive way than is possible through other research approaches. Internal surveys may also allow each member of an affected group to be involved in the strategic planning process, and to accomplish this participation in an equitable and consistent manner. External surveys have similar purposes. The advantages and disadvantages of telephone versus written surveys as information gathering techniques is best left to extended review in a market research book.[1]

Focus groups

This technique is the least frequently used of the three approaches, but growing more commonplace in strategic planning processes. Focus groups may be convened at any point in the process to gather information on a particular issue. Such groups are becoming a popular activity in the strategy formulation stage of the planning process and provide excellent forums for multidisciplinary development of strategy on a given issue. Here, too, the advantages and disadvantages of focus groups versus other research approaches is a larger subject than can be addressed here.[2]

Most strategic planning processes will employ more than one of the above approaches. And, with the growing recognition of the importance of a strong process in strategic planning, more extensive use of individual and multiple research approaches in strategic planning can be expected and should be encouraged in future planning efforts.

KEY STAKEHOLDER INVOLVEMENT

A brief review of the role and participation expectations for key stakeholder groups in the strategic planning process seems in order given the importance of superior planning process to the success of strategic planning.

Board members

The strategic planning committee is usually an ad hoc or standing committee of the board and, therefore, includes significant representation from this group. Board members will be important participants in retreats and subjects of internal research. The board should be concerned with the policy implication of strategic planning, and is generally and appropriately focused on the strategic direction portion of the strategic planning output.

Physicians

Physicians should be well represented on the strategic planning committee. They will often be the group that is the subject of the most extensive research of the internal (and sometimes external) constituencies. Physicians should be concerned with the clinical implications of strategic planning. Physicians may be most broadly affected by the outputs of the strategic planning process, but except in some of the emerging integrated delivery systems, they do not have direct approval authority or clear implementation responsibility.

Senior management

Senior management is almost always represented on the strategic planning committee, but is generally fewer in number and "voice" than either of the above groups. Management is the coordinator of the strategic planning process—structuring the process, staffing it, keeping it moving along, and overseeing implementation. Senior management's role and responsibilities in the planning process generally increase as the strategic planning process reaches its later stages.

Other clinicians

Depending on the nature of the organization, other clinicians (e.g., nurses, physical therapists, psychologists, etc.) may play a major or minor role in the strategic planning process. In healthcare organizations not dominated by hospitals or physicians, other clinicians may have significant involvement, including participation on the strategic planning committee of the board. In hospital- or physician-dominated healthcare organizations, other clinicians will play a minimal role or have no role in the strategic planning process, but will usually get involved when implementation nears.

Other management

In most cases, other management members only will get involved in the strategic planning process prior to implementation if a significant issue or area of concern arises over which they have direct responsibility or expertise. Although some strategic planning experts advocate a bottom-up strategic planning process, few healthcare organizations practice such an approach.

Notes

1. Alreck, P. L., and R. B. Settle. 1995. *The Survey Research Handbook.* Chicago: Irwin Professional Publishing.
2. Greenbaum, T. L. 1993. *The Handbook for Focus Group Research.* New York: Lexington Books.

CHAPTER 8

Case Study: St. David's Health Care System, Austin, Texas

S T. DAVID'S Health Care System (SDHCS) is typical, in many respects, of larger community hospitals that have prospered in the environment of the past 20 years. SDHCS has benefited further by virtue of its location in Austin, Texas, a rapidly growing state capital, a major university center (University of Texas), and the hub of an expanding industrial and high technology center.

During the period covered by the case study, 1984 through 1997, SDHCS grew from 313 beds to 438 beds and from approximately $40 million in annual revenues to $130 million. SDHCS's scope of services broadened considerably during this period; most notably, it added a broad range of psychiatry, physical medicine and rehabilitation services, and tertiary services, such as open-heart surgery. SDHCS is successfully transitioning from a fee-for-service environment to a highly managed environment. In 1996, managed care covered 65 percent of the population in Austin, and SDHCS derived 40 percent of its revenues from managed care in fiscal year 1996.

Unlike many other metropolitan areas, Austin has been and is expected to continue to experience rapid population growth. In 1980, the Austin metropolitan area had a population of about 540,000; it increased approximately 45 percent to 780,000 by 1990, and is expected to grow another 20 percent to nearly one million by the year 2000. In part because Austin is home to a large university, its population is younger than that of the state or nation as a whole. This factor and the high managed care penetration explain the relatively low use rates for expensive acute care services in the Austin metropolitan area.

The high growth rate and generally affluent population have attracted many competitors to the Austin area. As recently as 1995, there were 7 general acute care hospitals with 1,500 beds (excluding psychiatric and rehabilitation beds), and 5 psychiatric and rehabilitation hospitals with a total of about 700 beds; however, very little system development had occurred except for a minor presence of Columbia/HCA. In 1995–96, hospital system formation resulted in the consolidation of the acute care hospitals and most of the psychiatric and rehabilitation hospitals into two competing systems: a Catholic-sponsored system led by Seton Medical Center and including the publicly owned hospital, and a joint venture of SDHCS and Columbia/HCA.

This case study covers the 12-year period that preceded the collaboration of SDHCS and Columbia/HCA's Austin-area facilities and profiles an organization committed to ongoing strategic planning. Formal strategic plans were developed in 1984, 1988, and 1992 by SDHCS, and significant planning activities occurred in the intervening years, including regular updates of the previous plans. SDHCS used the strategic planning process to focus its planning and development activities, and derived many tangible benefits from the planning process and outputs as the planning chronology described below indicates.

1984 STRATEGIC PLAN

St. David's Health Care System, then known as St. David's Community Hospital (SDCH), began in 1983 the first of 3 eventual strategic plan development efforts over a 12-year period. In the spring of that year, with its major facility concerns being addressed in a renovation and expansion program, SDCH determined that a strategic planning process would allow the hospital to allocate its resources most effectively to meet the healthcare needs of the greater Austin community while maintaining a competitive position in the healthcare market. A comprehensive strategic planning process was initiated and featured extensive internal and external data analysis, primary market research involving medical staff and consumers, and development and evaluation of multiple future scenarios, which culminated in the selection of one composite scenario for the future role of the hospital.

The strategic planning process was initiated when the environment was being influenced by two major, interrelated themes: continuing inflation in healthcare costs was being recognized as a national problem and the implementation of the prospective payment system using diagnosis-related groups (DRGs) for inpatient care had commenced as a mechanism to effect some measure of cost control by the federal government. Other important issues influencing the potential future strategic direction for SDCH and other providers at that time included the explosion of technological advances and the increasing number and types of competitors entering the expanding healthcare industry, especially for-profit organizations. The planning analysis recognized that SDCH, and healthcare providers generally, were entering an era of increasingly rapid change, but the outlines of the future healthcare delivery system and the role of providers such as SDCH in the future system were, at best, hazy at that time.

After identifying and assessing six different future roles for SDCH, the strategic plan concluded that a combination of future roles offered the best alternative for SDCH's future development. It characterized this broader role as one of a "full-service community hospital offering select secondary and tertiary services," which also included:

- active participant in multi-institutional arrangements;
- diversified healthcare corporation (with a much broader program and service mix than inpatient medical and surgical, and obstetric care); and
- regional referral center competing with Seton Medical Center and Brackenridge Hospital, the other large hospitals located in Austin.

The strategic plan concluded with ten major recommendations for SDCH's future development:

Recommendation 1

St. David's Community Hospital should develop additional clinical programs. Those programs should include invasive cardiac services (cardiac catheterization services and open-heart surgery), an emergency department, rehabilitation services, and services for the elderly.

Recommendation 2

St. David's Community Hospital should expand and enhance existing services, particularly obstetrics, and develop selected centers of excellence.

Recommendation 3

St. David's Community Hospital should attract more physicians to its campus.

Recommendation 4

St. David's Community Hospital should participate in alternative delivery systems.

Recommendation 5

St. David's Community Hospital should develop programs for the major employers in the Austin area.

Recommendation 6

St. David's Community Hospital should intensify its marketing program, enhance the community's awareness of the hospital, and enhance the community's image of the hospital.

Recommendation 7

St. David's Community Hospital should participate in shared services opportunities and multi-institutional arrangements.

Recommendation 8

St. David's Community Hospital should add inpatient beds, as necessary, to serve expanded program needs and meet demand.

Recommendation 9

St. David's Community Hospital should revise its corporate structure to the degree necessary to accomplish these recommendations.

Recommendation 10

St. David's Community Hospital should change its name to reflect the broader geographic markets it will serve with the implementation of recommendations one through nine.

SDCH moved quickly from planning to implementation and in the next four years implemented nearly all aspects of the recommendations made and in some instances more. By 1988, the hospital was well on its way to repositioning itself as a regional healthcare system, equivalent in many respects to the two other large hospital and referral centers in Austin. Obstetric and cardiology services were true centers of excellence, and the construction of new pavilions for broad-based psychiatric and rehabilitation programs was well under way. In recognition of its expanded role, the organization was renamed St. David's Health Care System.

1988 STRATEGIC PLAN

SDHCS commenced the formal update of its strategic plan in March 1988. An underlying premise of the strategic planning process was that the regional healthcare environment within which SDHCS would operate would exemplify several major characteristics during the next five years, including:

- the demands for healthcare services will be dynamic and will continue to change;

- providers of healthcare services who are leaders in central Texas will be in the healthcare, rather than the traditional hospital, business; and
- the delivery of healthcare services will be influenced by the continued development and increased competitiveness of managed care systems.

The strategic planning process consisted of five activities:

- Activity I: Environmental assessment;
- Activity II: Goal formulation;
- Activity III: Strategy formulation;
- Activity IV: Identification of resource requirements; and
- Activity V: Strategic plan conclusions and recommendations.

This process is an earlier version of the strategic planning process described in previous chapters of this book. As in the 1984 strategic plan, the planning process included, in addition to the analytical work, interaction among senior SDHCS administrative staff and presentations to the planning committee of the board and the medical staff planning committee.

The environment in which SDHCS was operating in 1988 had evolved in a number of striking ways from that which was present at the outset of the 1984 strategic plan. Overall, providers in the Austin metropolitan area had progressed significantly from strategies predicated on the regulated era of healthcare to those of the evolving free market and emerging competitive era. Managed care had established itself as a force to be dealt with in the regional marketplace. SDHCS estimated that 10 percent of its total revenue in 1988 was derived from managed care organizations and the amount and proportion of total revenue represented by managed care companies was forecast to be the dominant reimbursement mechanism within the next decade.

As a result of this perspective on the environment and other aspects of external and internal situation, SDHCS identified six key planning issues. For each issue, a five-year goal and a series of implementing strategies and actions were delineated as summarized below.

Issue 1: Positioning for managed care products

SDHCS will maintain a managed care position that is at least equivalent to that of the organization's market position in nonmanaged care programs.

Issue 2: Adequate primary care physician referral base

SDHCS will maintain an adequate number and mix of primary care physicians whose practice locations are geographically dispersed throughout the system's regional service area in order to form a feeder network and maintain sufficient referrals to specialists.

Issue 3: Medical staff bonding and recruitment

SDHCS will increase loyalties of existing medical staff, selectively develop new loyalties, and continue to be positioned as the most physician-oriented hospital in the region.

Issue 4: Optimal program and service mix

SDHCS will operate competitive and efficient services. It will operate at 80 percent occupancy of its existing acute care beds, and 80 and 85 percent respectively of new 80-bed and 107-bed psychiatric and re-habilitation and skilled nursing facilities. Comprehensive ambulatory care services, efficiently organized, will be provided as a complement to medical staff services to serve the needs of SDHCS's regional service area.

Issue 5: Relationship with hospitals in outlying areas (networking)

SDHCS will employ hospital networking as one method to gain increasing control of tertiary care referrals and develop mutually beneficial relationships with hospitals in central Texas and their staffs whose culture, mission, and service mix are compatible with those of SDHCS.

Issue 6: Organization, operations, and finance

SDHCS developed seven goals relating to governance and administrative effectiveness, improvement of campus access and traffic flow, and maintenance of financially prudent operations.

As was the case in the 1984 plan, SDHCS moved rapidly from planning to implementation. It largely accomplished the goals, strategies, and actions in the 1988 plan by 1992 with the exception of those related to issue 5, hospital networking. The management team's assessment of the lack of progress in hospital networking was that the rural hospitals in the region were still doing fairly well financially and did not see the need for formal relationships with SDHCS or others at that time. Despite the best efforts of SDHCS's executive team, little was accomplished in this area between 1988 and 1992. With the rest of the strategies in the 1988 plan essentially completed or well under way, by 1992 it was time to update the strategic plan once again.

1992 STRATEGIC PLAN

The 1992 update of the SDHCS strategic plan was initiated when federal healthcare reform was anticipated. The planning process was carried out during the election campaign and national debate on what to do about the U.S. healthcare system. Discussion naturally focused on 2 principal issues: how to control seemingly limitless, double-digit increases in healthcare costs, and what to do about the approximately 40 million Americans who had no health insurance. Much local debate centered on how these issues might be addressed and what implications resolving these issues would have for SDHCS.

Other major environmental influences affecting the potential plans for SDHCS in 1992 were:

- continued rapid population growth in the Austin metro area;
- significant and increasing managed care penetration in the area;
- emerging recognition of physician oversupply, especially in sub-specialty disciplines;
- technology advances and payment changes spurring the growth of outpatient services;
- the end of certificate-of-need regulatory constraints in Texas leading to a flourishing, competitive market; and
- the potential for competition based on real quality differences in the not-too-distant future as indicated by patient satisfaction measurement and rudimentary technical quality assessment efforts.

These environmental influences had a major impact on the plans and strategies that SDHCS would develop, and also had a direct effect on the nature of the process used to develop the strategic plan. In particular, the degree of uncertainty about the future environment suggested that a more inclusive planning process, with greater and more frequent participation from important SDHCS constituencies than had occurred in the past, would be appropriate. While the major difference from prior planning efforts was in the amount and type of physician participation in the process, there was also more extensive and frequent interaction among the board, the board planning committee, and the management staff of SDHCS. In addition to individual and group physician interviews and meetings, a medical staff planning committee was convened and met a number of times during the process. This group provided a forum for focused physician participation, including review of issues and potential alternative courses for addressing the issues. This group also served as a communications channel to the medical staff as a whole. Figures 8.1 and 8.2 illustrate the substantive strategic planning activities and the role of leadership groups in the planning process.

The core output of the strategic planning process is SDHCS's mission, vision, and goals, summarized in Figure 8.3. To meet the

Figure 8.1 Strategic Planning Process

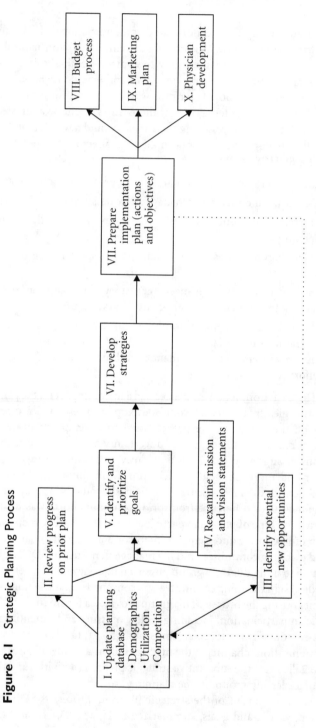

Source: St. David's Health Care System, 1992.

Figure 8.2 Planning Process Tasks and Responsibilities

Tasks

I. Update planning
database

II. Review progress on prior plan
III. Identify potential new opportunities
IV. Reexamine mission and vision statements
V. Identify and prioritize goals
VI. Develop strategies

VII. Prepare implementation plan
(actions and objectives)
VIII. Budget process
IX. Marketing plan
X. Physician development

Responsibilities

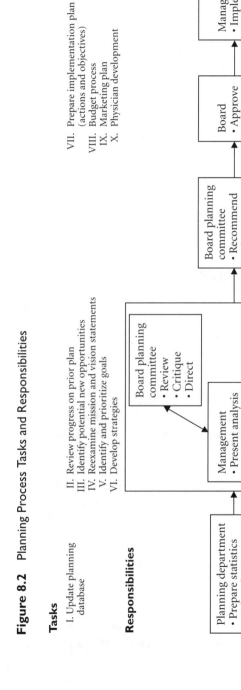

Source: St. David's Health Care System, 1992.

challenges of the emerging healthcare environment, SDHCS saw the benefit of developing a vertically integrated system. As one of the two most formidable healthcare organizations in the Austin area at the time, SDHCS believed that it could dictate, to a large degree, its own destiny and form an integrated delivery system. With a number of years of solid financial performance behind it, a strong and supportive medical staff, and high customer and managed care plan satisfaction, SDHCS believed it had the strength to be a leader and a catalyst in the metropolitan area market, emerging as the flagship that would dominate the Austin area healthcare delivery system entering the twenty-first century.

Although elements of the plan's strategy were extremely visionary and farsighted in orientation, the organization recognized that its long-term future would not be realized without continuing solid short-term and medium-term performance. Many of the goals and accompanying objectives and actions addressed these needs directly through initiatives aimed at core inpatient services, emerging specialty areas of emphasis, the growing ambulatory care sector, and creative and systematic value enhancement.

ST. DAVID'S HEALTH CARE SYSTEM TODAY

As in previous strategic plan implementation efforts, SDHCS moved quickly and purposefully to operationalize the 1992 strategic plan update. Good progress was made on all fronts and many of the goals were well on their way to being achieved within the defined five-year time frame.

The Austin metropolitan area market evolved as anticipated in 1992, except, of course, for the failure of national healthcare reform. While the general direction of marketplace evolution was consistent with the perspective of the future environment formulated in 1992, the specifics of market evolution were somewhat different than anticipated. And while the 1992 strategic plan correctly forecast the kinds of changes that have occurred (managed care growth, declining inpatient utilization, accelerating financial pressures), the intensity of the changes and relentless pressures on providers have proven to be even more onerous than imagined at that time.

In response to the intense changes, more horizontal integration activity has occurred. Two major stimulants for this have been the unforeseen difficulties encountered by the large public hospital in Austin, Brackenridge Hospital, which ultimately led to the county deciding to lease it on a long-term basis to Seton Medical Center, SDHCS's major competitor. Also during this period, Columbia/HCA

Figure 8.3 St. David's Health Care System

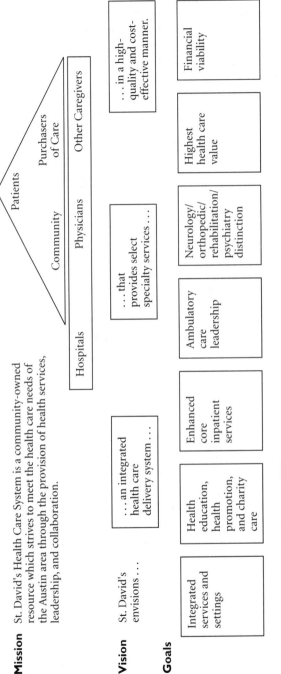

Mission St. David's Health Care System is a community-owned resource which strives to meet the health care needs of the Austin area through the provision of health services, leadership, and collaboration.

Vision St. David's envisions . . .

. . . an integrated health care delivery system . . .

. . . that provides select specialty services . . .

. . . in a high-quality and cost-effective manner.

Hospitals Community Physicians Purchasers of Care Other Caregivers Patients

Goals

Integrated services and settings

Health education, health promotion, and charity care

Enhanced core inpatient services

Ambulatory care leadership

Neurology/ orthopedic/ rehabilitation/ psychiatry distinction

Highest health care value

Financial viability

Source: St. David's Health Care System, 1992.

emerged as a major national force and as a major force in the Austin marketplace. To counter the Seton-Brackenridge alliance, SDHCS and Columbia/HCA formed a partnership in the Austin metropolitan area, each contributing their three hospitals to form a new system jointly owned and operated by the two organizations.

The new system is still young and its future direction is not yet clear. However, given the history and success of SDHCS in the Austin-area marketplace, it is reasonable to imagine that yet another update of the SDHCS strategic plan will begin shortly, to chart a course that will serve the new system well as it enters the twenty-first century.

CHAPTER 9

Case Study: Wayne General Hospital, Wayne, New Jersey

Justin E. Doheny and Alan M. Zuckerman

HISTORICAL BACKGROUND · · · · · · · · · · ·

WAYNE GENERAL Hospital originally opened in 1871 as Ladies Hospital in Paterson, New Jersey. Established by a Protestant women's group to care for the poor, the hospital prospered as Paterson's manufacturing industry, particularly textiles, thrived. With the invention of nylon in the 1940s and the migration of the textile industry to the Carolinas, Paterson fell into economic decline. The hospital, then known as Paterson General Hospital, was also hard hit.

The turmoil of the 1960s further aggravated Paterson's economic outlook. The once well-respected hospital was now faced with aging facilities and outdated services, operating in a region plagued by poverty and an excess of acute care hospitals. In 1966, the leaders of Paterson General Hospital elected to abandon their urban roots and relocate to the suburbs. Land was purchased in nearby Wayne, New Jersey, with plans to partner with an adjacent state college to develop a medical and nursing school. The hospital's name was changed to Greater Paterson General Hospital to reflect its new service area.

Angry at the departure of the hospital, the mayor of Paterson and the area's competing hospitals successfully sued to block the closure of the hospital's facilities, and Greater Paterson General was forced to operate in both Wayne and Paterson. Financial pressures from serving both areas drove the hospital into bankruptcy, from which it emerged in 1975. The bankruptcy court required that the hospital continue to operate a primary care clinic in Paterson, pay a monthly fee to the remaining hospitals, and accept ambulance patients from one-third of the districts in the city, including some of the city's poorest residents. Nonetheless, the move to Wayne had proceeded, and in 1973, the new facilities were opened on a 70-acre wooded tract.

In 1978, the hospital was included in New Jersey's DRG re-imbursement experiment. With its historic costs, which had been artificially depressed due to bankruptcy, a major factor in calculation of its rate base, the DRG experiment would hamper the hospital's fiscal health until the conclusion of the experiment in 1993. In 1983, the hospital changed its name to Wayne General Hospital in an effort to broaden its appeal to a more affluent, suburban market and to distance itself from its historic urban setting.

In 1984, a major expansion project was initiated to enlarge selected support and clinical areas. Financial constraints experienced during the move from Paterson had forced the hospital to downsize its original construction plans for the new facility, and expansion was now necessary; the significant new debt for the expansion, however, was assumed without any easily identifiable sources of added revenue.

In 1986, the first of the hospital's most recent vintage of strategic plans was completed. The plan included two major initiatives: the construction of an ambulatory care center in the northern part of the county and development of a geriatric program. Following the collapse of the real estate market in northern New Jersey, and the slowdown in suburban development and population growth, the ambulatory care center initiative was abandoned in 1987. The geriatric program has gradually expanded into a broad range of programs for seniors in the hospital's service area.

By the summer of 1992, the hospital's management team, and eventually the board and medical staff, recognized the inevitable shakeout that would occur among local hospitals. They approached a neighboring hospital to discuss the potential benefits of a merger. After a six-month effort led by consultants, the two hospitals were unable to agree on a governance plan. The long history of competition between the hospitals could not be overcome and an intractable rift emerged.

Recognizing the impact of this setback in the spring of 1993, the leadership of Wayne General Hospital decided that the organization needed a solid plan of action to cope with the vast uncertainties in its operating environment. Until 1993, New Jersey hospitals operated under a highly regulated reimbursement system. A deregulated system planned for 1994 was expected to accelerate the shift to managed care and increase competition. In the hospital's market of Wayne and other northeastern New Jersey communities, competitors had begun discussing partnerships with other providers to respond to managed care initiatives and cope with excess capacity.

With occupancy dropping from 90 percent in 1989 to 79 percent in 1992, and an average length of stay that increased from 6.2 in 1989 to 7.9 in 1992, Wayne General Hospital was concerned about competition and managed care. How would the hospital anticipate and adapt to the new incentives and penalties of a managed care system? How would physicians be integrated into the delivery system? How would the hospital reposition itself in the nonacute and outpatient business? How would resources be managed to ensure high-value medical care?

THE 1994 STRATEGIC PLAN

In September 1993, Wayne General Hospital formally initiated strategic planning. The plan was slated to address three major issues:

- What will the northern New Jersey market look like?
- What roles can Wayne General play in the market? What role should it play?
- What steps need to be taken now—both internally (within Wayne General Hospital) and externally (market interface)?

Guided by a master planning committee that included members of the board, medical staff, and administration, the planning process included four activities, shown in Figure 9.1, including situation analysis, strategic direction, strategy formulation, and action planning.

Activity I: Situation Analysis

The situation analysis examined Wayne General Hospital's internal and external operating environment including historical utilization, financial data, medical staff trends, facilities and equipment, competencies and vulnerabilities, demographic and economic trends, and competitors. Over 40 interviews with the hospital's management team, physicians, board members, and external parties were conducted to gather information about market and organization dynamics. A written survey of the entire medical staff was also completed.

The analysis revealed that Wayne General Hospital had a 16 percent marketshare in its primary service area and a 6 percent share in its secondary area, with population growth in both areas

Figure 9.1 The Strategic Planning Process

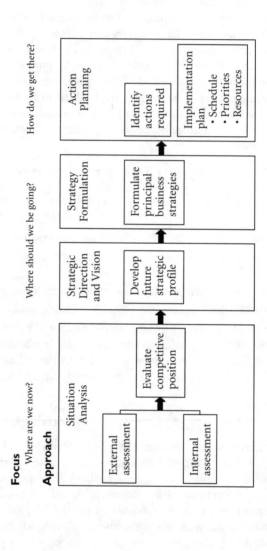

Source: Wayne General Hospital, 1994.

stagnant. Inpatient discharges had declined in recent years, and were projected to continue to fall. Admission rates were over 130 per 1,000 population in New Jersey and 145 at Wayne General in 1993, but heavily managed markets were exhibiting admissions at under 100 per 1,000 population, translating into a projected need of 20 to 50 percent fewer inpatient beds in three to five years. Wayne General Hospital's average length of stay (ALOS) and utilization rates were also high compared to national and regional averages, and much higher than in heavily managed markets.

In terms of ambulatory care volumes, Wayne General Hospital lagged behind most U.S. hospitals. In 1990, outpatient revenue was 22 percent of the hospital's total revenue, but dropped to 17.5 percent in 1993. Despite a lack of growth in outpatient volume, the hospital's financial position improved substantially during this time period. After several years of negative operating performance, the hospital's operating margin was 3.8 percent in 1993, exceeding the 3 percent considered the minimum for annual replacement and expansion of the plant and equipment. Liquidity had also improved, and was better than most of the hospital's competitors; however, a lack of capital reserves made operating performance a concern, and precluded assumption of debt for capital expenditures.

Wayne General Hospital's medical staff was dominated by solo practice physicians, which is the least desirable practice model for managed care. At a time when one-third of all physicians were in group practice, and at higher rates in heavily managed markets, 70 percent of Wayne General Hospital's staff were in solo practice. The staff was also older than at comparable hospitals and lacked the primary care physicians needed in the next five years. While the hospital was ahead of its competitors in PHO development, many physicians indicated that Wayne General Hospital was their second-choice hospital.

The medical staff was fairly positive in their assessment of the hospital's management team that had been in place about five years, but less supportive of the board. The 24-member board was larger than the national average of 14, and lacked representation from key corporations in the area. There were also no limits on terms of service on the board.

The situation analysis was distilled into a SWOTs assessment that served as the basis for Activity III discussions about strategic direction:

Strengths

Strengths included geographic location, strong (recent) operating performance, geriatric services, high occupancy rate, and PHO development.

Weaknesses

Weaknesses included heavy indigent care responsibility, lack of distinctive services, obstetrics, pediatrics, emergency services, medical staff organization, lack of capital, declining volumes, low case-mix index, no national affiliation, and freestanding community hospital.

Opportunities

Opportunities included networks and affiliations, expense and ALOS reduction, hospital-physician coordination, medical staff development, nonacute service development, increased penetration of the primary service area, and increased board effectiveness.

Threats

Threats included exclusion from managed care contracts, shrinking acute market, being forced to remain freestanding, and limited reimbursement.

Activity II: Strategic Direction

To establish strategic direction for the hospital, the planning committee reviewed the key strategic issues facing the hospital and analyzed alternative future scenarios that could occur as the hospital attempted to address these issues. The scenarios were evaluated to determine the optimal future direction for the hospital. The direction was then summarized in a vision statement describing what the organization wished to become in the next ten years:

> Wayne General Hospital intends to be a community-oriented healthcare center providing a broad range of integrated primary and secondary care services effectively linked to other healthcare providers who complement and support the services we offer. We intend our organization to be distinguished by the diversity, quality, and cost-effectiveness of our services. Through growth in ambulatory care and nonacute care, we expect to be a more diverse and vital healthcare organization.

Next, a planning conference was convened with representatives of the board, medical staff, and senior management to review progress and gain input on strategic direction and strategies. Five key strategies emerged from discussions at the planning conference:

1. The hospital must attain a low-cost position in the market.
2. The hospital must become a "managed care friendly" organization.

3. Nonacute care development must occur soon.

4. The hospital must be aggressive in medical staff development.

5. Affiliation exploration must occur.

Activity III: Strategy Formulation

With overall organization direction and strategies defined, the hospital appointed a task force for each of the five strategies. These groups were charged with translating the key strategies into tangible, intermediate and short-term positions and actions for the hospital. For each strategy, a goal describing the desired position of the hospital by 1999 was developed. Rationales for the goals were then developed, and objectives for the first year were delineated. A summary of the goals and objectives is presented below.

Strategy 1

- **Goal:** By 1999, the hospital will have a lower cost per case and per day than its major competitors, without compromising quality. A similar position will be attained for nonacute services.

- **Objective:** Wayne General Hospital completes a major operations improvement project.

Strategy 2

- **Goal:** The hospital and its medical staff are successful in attaining every managed care contract sought.

- **Objective:** Wayne General Hospital increases its percentage of revenue received from managed care payors to 10.8 percent in 1994 and 16.3 percent in 1995, from 5.5 percent in 1993.

Strategy 3

- **Goal:** The hospital receives 50 percent of its gross revenue from nonacute care services (or expenses under a capitated system) with specific improvements in the emergency department; ambulatory surgery and other outpatient services; nursing home, subacute care, and assisted living; and home health.

- **Objective:** Revenue from nonacute services increases 20 percent annually from increased utilization.

Strategy 4

- **Goal:** Wayne General Hospital's medical staff will be composed principally of primary care physicians who are leaders in providing primary care and secondary care in the region.

- **Objective:** The hospital establishes contracts with outside organizations using its PHO; the PHO forms a group of at least 15 primary care physicians and provides management services organization (MSO) functions to interested physicians.

Strategy 5

- **Goal:** The hospital plays a central role as a community healthcare organization in a provider and insurer network that is one of the two or three dominant delivery systems in northern New Jersey.
- **Objective:** Affiliation discussions are underway or completed.

Under Strategy 5, the hospital also laid out purposes of affiliation (rationale for why the organization wants to affiliate) and criteria for affiliation (indicators to measure the probability of a successful affiliation), which are presented in Figures 9.2 and 9.3.

Activity V: Action Planning

To assist with the tracking of implementation activities, a list of first-year actions was developed and plotted on a matrix to show how the actions correlated to the five key strategies (see Table 9.1). Next, an implementation plan was developed that listed major actions required for each strategy, and the associated time frame and estimated resource requirements. This plan was a fluid document that was modified as the individuals responsible for implementation became more involved in the process. Wayne General Hospital's implementation plan for the cost reduction strategy (Strategy 1) is presented in Table 9.2.

RESULTS OF 1994 STRATEGIC PLAN

Wayne General Hospital has made great strides in implementing the five major strategies that emerged from the formal planning process. To address the Strategy 1 goal of improving cost competitiveness, the hospital formed a multidisciplinary task force, composed of physicians and hospital staff, to lead an operations improvement effort. Improvements thus far include a reduction in medical and surgical length of stay by 2.45 days, implementation of a case management system with active physician involvement, elimination of delays in discharge planning, and improvement in turnaround times in selected ancillary departments. Development of a clinical cost-accounting system enabled the hospital to improve cost management and track patient utilization and costs across ancillary departments and for routine care. Reengineering in several departments also improved operational efficiency.

Figure 9.2 Purposes of Affiliation for Wayne General Hospital

Primary
- Access to managed care contracts
- Economies of scale and cost competitiveness
  - Purchasing
  - Shared services
  - Cost-effective utilization of technology
- Ability to participate in development of successful integrated delivery system

Secondary
- Assistance in program development
- Assistance in medical staff development
- Access to capital for Wayne General Hospital
- Enhanced prestige
- Statewide clout

Source: Wayne General Hospital, 1994.

Strategy 2 was successfully addressed with more aggressive contracting efforts coordinated with the officers of the PHO. By the end of 1995, more than 17 percent of the hospital's revenue was from managed care and 37 contracts were in place. Following the completion of an affiliation agreement, contracts with market leader managed care organizations were obtained, and Wayne General Hospital is now on its way to sustaining a managed care revenue stream that is superior to its nearest competitors.

A number of activities have been completed or are underway to achieve the Strategy 3 goal of increasing the hospital's revenue from nonacute care services. A certificate of need to establish a freestanding ambulatory surgery center with the hospital's physicians has been approved. Construction of a new endoscopic procedure room and mammography suite is now complete. An adult day care program has been developed in Wayne, and a 300-unit continuing care retirement community is being pursued with Marriott. In addition, a certificate-of-need application for a 14-bed hospital-based subacute care unit has been approved, and a certificate of need to renovate and expand the emergency room has been submitted.

To increase the number and quality of primary care physicians on the hospital's medical staff, as stated in Strategy 4, Wayne General Hospital has developed a primary care acquisition strategy, and has targeted four practices loyal to the hospital for recruitment.

Figure 9.3 Criteria for Successful Affiliation for Wayne General Hospital

---

Medical Staff
- **Relationships.** Do our physicians refer to physicians at the hospital? If not, would they?
- **Quality.** Are their doctors of the quality we want to associate with and refer to?
- **Range.** Does the hospital and its medical staff offer essentially all of the services we might require in caring for our patients?

Patients
- **Relationships.** Do our patients currently go to the hospital for any services? Would our patients follow physician referrals to the hospital?

Governance
- **Philosophy and Mission.** Do we have consistent philosophies and missions?
- **Image.** Is this a hospital with which we want to associate? How will the community view the affiliation?
- **Autonomy.** How much local autonomy can be retained?
- **Stability.** Is the potential affiliate a stable business?
- **Compatibility.** Are the organizations compatible overall?

Administration
- **Compatibility.** How compatible are the management staffs? Will day-to-day interactions be easy?
- **Range.** Does the hospital offer the support we need or might need?

Source: Wayne General Hospital, 1994.

The hospital is also helping physicians gain access to managed care contracts and has forged a partnership with a large physician group in northern New Jersey. In conjunction with a systemwide physician integration strategy, the hospital is assisting with the management of the Wayne General Physician-Hospital Organization and the Wayne General Independent Practice Association.

The final strategy of the 1994 strategic plan addressed the hospital's need to affiliate to ensure participation in one of the dominant delivery systems in northern New Jersey. The hospital conducted a strategic and financial analysis of 18 potential partners across northern New Jersey and the New York City metropolitan area using the criteria detailed in Figure 9.3. With guidance from a task force of trustees, medical staff leaders, management, and attending physicians, the 18 candidates were ranked and site visits were conducted

Table 9.1 Matrix of One-Year Actions Relative to the Five Key Strategies

Actions	Key Strategies				
	Cost Competitiveness	Managed Care	Markets and Programs	Medical Staff	Affiliation
Increase productivity, improve systems in the hospital	●	■	●		
Develop protocols for quality improvement/length-of-stay reduction	●	■	■	●	■
Audit information systems capabilities	●	●			■
Develop ambulatory services strategy		■	●		
Upgrade obstetrics program		●	●	■	
Improve emergency services delivery			●	■	
Evaluate feasibility of other nonacute services	■		●		■
Sign managed care contracts and develop pricing strategies		●	●	■	■
Facilitate group formation		■		●	
Assist and develop primary care network		■		●	■
Develop practice succession and transitioning program				●	
Improve physician-hospital cohesiveness		●		■	
Conduct baseline community health assessment		■	●		■
Improve and develop marketing program		■	●		
Assess and develop affiliations	■	■	■	■	●

Key:
● = Action best fits under this strategy.
■ = Action is applicable to this strategy but is addressed under a different strategy in the text.
Source: Wayne General Hospital, 1994.

Table 9.2   Implementation Plan for Wayne General Hospital

Category/Action	Estimated Expense Responsibility: Ms. YX		Calendar Year				
COST REDUCTION	Capital	Operating	1994	1995	1996	1997	1998
Undergo length-of-stay reduction program • Expand case-management program	Low	Low	▬	▬			
• Develop and implement at least ten clinical care pathways per year	Low	Low	▬	▬	▬	▬	▬
• Identify ways to move patients to most appropriate (nonacute care) settings					▬	▬	
Reengineer patient care delivery systems to increase productivity and reduce labor cost		Medium	▬	▬	▬		
Implement information systems plan with particular focus on: • Cost-accounting system	High	Low	▬	▬			
• Operating room scheduling	Medium		▬	▬			
• Materials management	Low		▬	▬			
Provide ongoing professional education to medical staff, nursing staff, and other patient care staff regarding resource utilization		Low	▬	▬	▬	▬	▬
Analyze physician utilization of ancillary services and devise a method to provide the physicians with price alerts on charges for services being ordered		Low	▬	▬			
Establish physician mentor program to help guide "high-cost" physicians toward cost-effective clinical choices		Low		▬	▬		

Key:

    Low = Less than $100,000
    Medium = $100,000 to $500,000
    High = More than $500,000
Source: Wayne General Hospital, 1994.

at the top 5 organizations. Following a poll of the medical staff, the board, management, and medical staff agreed to initiate affiliation discussions with the candidate ranked second by the task force, and first among the medical staff.

Negotiations proceeded over a six-month period, but ultimately broke down over issues of governance and control. The remaining four potential partners were reevaluated, and in September 1995, negotiations with Saint Barnabas Medical Center in Livington, New Jersey, were recommended. Negotiations were initiated in December 1995 and concluded by February 1996. The new Saint Barnabas Health Care System was formed in May 1996 with the consolidation of the parent holding companies of eight hospitals across New Jersey. Wayne General Hospital is now a charter member of the largest system in the state.

CHAPTER 10

Case Study:
Post-Acute Services

Karl G. Bartscht

SUCCESSFUL INTEGRATED delivery systems will provide or have access to a full continuum of care for the covered lives they serve. One frequently overlooked component of the continuum, and one with significant cost savings and revenue enhancement potential, is post-acute care. Without access to post-acute services, patients remain in costly acute care settings when downstaging to a less costly setting is more appropriate. As a result, healthcare organizations lose billions of dollars each year on excess inpatient days for which they receive no reimbursement.

The flow of patients through the post-acute continuum is illustrated in Figure 10.1. Though current reimbursement generally requires an acute hospital stay prior to admission to a post-acute setting, in the future, more patients will be admitted directly to post-acute settings. Currently, approximately 20 percent of acute medical and surgical patients are discharged to post-acute services, excluding home health services.[1] However, as lengths of stay continue to shorten and patients are discharged earlier in the recovery phase, an increasing number of patients will be candidates for some level of post-acute services, including acute rehabilitation, long-term care hospital, home health, skilled nursing facility, subacute care, adult medical day care, and assisted living.

Aggressively managed care and the increased availability of post-acute services will lead to reduction of acute care beds from the

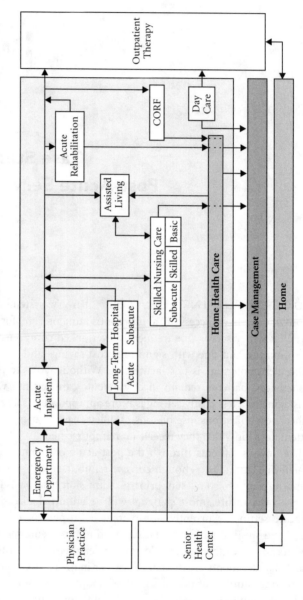

Figure 10.1 Flow of Patients within a Continuum of Case Management (Acute, Post-Acute, and Subacute Care)

Source: Chi Systems, Inc., 1997.

current level of 2.5 beds per 1,000 population to as low as 1 bed per 1,000 population. As care in managed health plans becomes aggressively managed, acute care days will drop almost 60 percent while subacute days will increase 47 percent and home health care visits will increase 17 percent.[2] Figure 10.2 illustrates the change in utilization of selected services as the healthcare environment evolves from a loosely managed, through a moderately managed, to an aggressively managed model.

The impact post-acute care will have on healthcare is even more dramatic when expenditures are viewed on a national level. In 1994, post-acute services accounted for 11 percent of the $949.4 billion total of national healthcare expenditures. Projections for 2010 estimate $3.4 trillion in healthcare expenditures, with post-acute

Figure 10.2 Post-Acute Bed and Visit Utilization of 100,000 Covered Lives

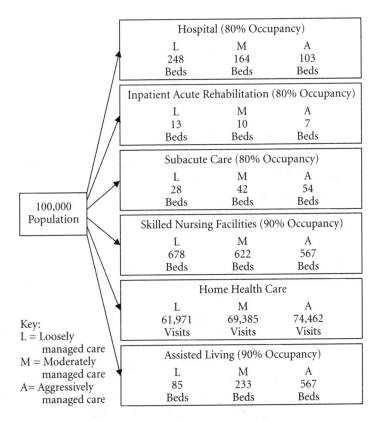

Source: Chi Systems, Inc., 1997.

services composing about 26 percent of the expenditures.[3] Astute organizations will anticipate the growth in this sector of the industry and be positioned to respond to market demands.

Currently, post-acute care is defined to include services that occur after an acute hospital stay. Elements of the post-acute services continuum include acute rehabilitation, long-term care hospital (a Medicare designation), skilled nursing facility (nursing home), subacute (which can include subunits within any of the previous services), assisted living, CORF (also a Medicare designation), day care, and home health care.

POST-ACUTE CARE STRATEGIC PLANNING

Strategic planning for post-acute care proceeds along the general steps outlined in previous chapters of this book. In each activity, there are, however, special characteristics that must be considered.

Activity I: Situation Analysis

The internal assessment identifies which post-acute services are currently being provided by the organization, as well as the demand for services generated by internal discharges. Physician and hospital staff (e.g., case managers, post-acute providers) interviews help identify options and barriers for the transfer of patients to post-acute services. Analysis of discharges by DRG determines length of stay versus benchmarks (e.g., the Medicare geometric mean), financial losses resulting from excess stays, and discharge destinations. Interviews and analysis of discharge data also help identify providers meeting current demand.

The external assessment identifies market characteristics and dynamics, and evaluates competitors' strengths and weaknesses. Market dynamics can have a dramatic impact on post-acute utilization, for example:

- With the rapid growth in the elderly population, it is projected that 5.3 million older adults will need nursing home care by 2030,[4] up from 1.5 million in 1990.[5]
- The use of skilled nursing–based intensive medical and rehabilitation units as primary referral sites for Medicare and Medicaid risk HMO patients will increase the demand for subacute beds.
- Subacute care has provided the springboard for future growth of the long-term care industry. Nursing home companies, once solely providers of routine geriatric care, are increasingly important providers in the overall continuum of care.

- Increased demand for rehabilitation has been fueled by reimbursement incentives, technological advances, and an aging population with a high incidence of chronic conditions.
- Case management will become care management. HMOs and capitated providers will identify their high-risk and chronic condition enrollees and place them under continuous care management, which will become the mechanism for patient placement.

A key output of the environmental assessment is quantification of demand for post-acute services generated by discharges from the acute care organization, as well as demand generated by the entire market. Providers currently meeting post-acute care demand will also be identified, and competitive positions will be described.

Activity II: Strategic Direction

This activity produces a strategic profile that emerges upon examining alternative futures, reassessing the organization's mission, establishing a vision for post-acute services, and developing key strategies.

Strategic planning for post-acute care must include a review of the organization's mission and vision to determine if the provision of post-acute services is appropriate. The organization must ask Are we in the healthcare delivery business? If not, Are we willing to be an acute inpatient care provider for a larger, integrated organization? These questions should be answered in light of the environmental assessment.

Considerations in developing mission and vision statements include:

- Do we ensure the availability of all post-acute services to our acute patients?
- What percentage of the market do we want to satisfy?
- Do we provide all post-acute services directly, do we offer access through strategic relations, or a combination of these?

The vision must be supported by strategies for development and provision of post-acute services, and should address the following considerations.

Make or buy

Although there may be significant opportunities for increased revenues and reduced costs, realizing these opportunities may require capital investment for acquisition, renovation, and new construction. Thus, availability of capital may limit initiatives, and may necessitate partnering to deliver certain post-acute services.

Reimbursement

As utilization of post-acute services increases, cost control pressures may also increase. Strategies must anticipate reimbursement changes.

Regulation

Because development of new post-acute services may be subject to certificate-of-need requirements, with subsequent operations regulated by state and federal certification processes, strategies must consider regulatory requirements.

Competition

Although all components of the post-acute continuum may be available in the market, some providers may not meet acceptable quality and access criteria. Those that do may be candidates for joint ventures.

Medical staff

In most cases, patients will be downstaged in the post-acute continuum by physician orders. Therefore, physicians must be involved in development of the continuum and educated on the appropriateness of post-acute settings.

Case management

The success of the post-acute continuum primarily hinges on the provision of a case (care) management program that ensures the appropriateness and timeliness of patient transfer.

Activity III: Strategy Formulation

Activity III of the planning process establishes goals and objectives for post-acute care services, as illustrated by the following case study.

The Saints Health System (SHS), a five-hospital healthcare system serving a metropolitan region, established the goal of being an integrated health system with the capability of serving one million covered lives. The SHS three-year strategic plan identified strategies and implementation steps by year. The plan states that a health system "must consist not only of traditional inpatient and outpatient activities, but also present the capability to provide those 'alternative' care options necessary to complete the health continuum."

In 1996, SHS leadership determined that development of the post-acute continuum represented a significant opportunity for the system, and that a post-acute services strategic plan should be prepared. Opportunities identified for post-acute services development included:

- unreimbursed costs of $36.5 million annually for excess lengths of stays that could be reduced by effective case management and facilitated by a complete post-acute continuum;
- opportunities to gain $38 million annually by providing post-acute services to SHS patients as well as the potential to expand services to other markets;
- opportunities to be on the cutting edge in responding to managed care initiatives; and
- the ability to provide the most effective continuum of healthcare.

To define the internal demand generated by the system for post-acute services, discharges were analyzed by DRG, and SHS physicians and hospital staff were interviewed. A total of 40,700 medical or surgical cases accounted for 256,400 patient days for an ALOS of 6.3 days. A total of 17,600 cases extended beyond the Medicare geometric mean by an average of 5 days. The analysis indicated the need for the following post-acute resources:

- Subacute beds at 90 percent occupancy—169
- Long-term care hospital beds at 90 percent occupancy—45
- Total potential rehabilitation candidates—588
- Total CORF visits—42,040

Physician interviews explored perceptions regarding delays in discharging patients, causes for the delays, availability and adequacy of post-acute services, and the types of post-acute clinical programs needed in the SHS. Interview results corroborated the post-acute needs analysis.

A market assessment determined the post-acute services market for SHS. An inventory of current services and volume generated by these services was completed. An analysis of potential affiliates was conducted to determine demand for post-acute services. Post-acute service demand for SHS was then identified for loose, moderate, and aggressive levels of managed care. SHS currently operates in a loosely to moderately penetrated managed care market, but with little real impact on the management of care. Projections (assuming for 296,000 covered lives) indicated a decrease in medical and surgical bed need from 533 (loosely managed) to 223 (aggressively managed), and a decrease in inpatient rehabilitation bed need from 39 to 22. These decreases would be offset by major increases in subacute and assisted living bed need, as well as an even greater increase in home health visits.

The final step was a thorough competitive assessment. Many post-acute services were not currently being provided (e.g., subacute) or were limited (e.g., long-term care hospital), so there was relatively little competition. It was determined that if SHS provided or had access to a full post-acute continuum, it could exercise significant control over patients directly discharged to these services. It was also determined that SHS's major competitors were enhancing their post-acute services.

The major competitors for post-acute services were 14 rehabilitation hospitals and hospital-based rehabilitation programs in SHS's four-county market area. In spite of these competitors, SHS was serving a larger share of the market, as measured by a combined inpatient census at their three inpatient rehabilitation programs, than did any of the competing hospitals.

SHS had been unable to open a skilled nursing facility because of certificate-of-need restrictions. However, many nursing homes were found to depend on SHS for transfer of patients, which could be the basis for future joint ventures or other opportunities.

Considerations in developing a post-acute continuum at SHS included:

- opportunities for enhancing case management and the potential to reduce acute patient stay;
- the potential to develop a long-term care hospital of 35 to 50 beds;
- the need for, and financial benefit of, developing subacute services at each of the SHS hospitals and nursing homes;
- barriers to subacute development, especially the moratorium on obtaining a license for skilled beds;
- the need to develop a nursing home network strategy to satisfy demand for both subacute and nursing home beds;
- the importance of establishing assisted living services as an alternative to nursing home beds;
- the large and growing need for home care services; and
- an opportunity to develop a continuum of physical medicine and rehabilitation services.

It was determined that SHS could benefit by almost $38 million annually in reduced costs or additional reimbursement by developing a complete post-acute continuum. The greatest returns were found to be in subacute care and long-term care hospital services. The total continuum could generate $145 million annually in revenues, but also would require capital investments in excess of $100 million. Because more than half of the capital would go to acquire nursing home beds, joint ventures and strategic alliances were recommended to develop a nursing home network, thereby reducing capital requirements.

Specific program actions recommended as part of the post-acute strategic plan included:

- enhancing and integrating case management activities to build a systemwide case management model;
- developing a long-term care hospital at one of the system's hospitals;
- developing subacute units at all hospitals and SHS-owned nursing homes and establishing joint venture subacute units at selected other nursing homes;
- devising a skilled nursing bed acquisition/joint venture/alliance strategy to ensure SHS access to high-quality nursing home care;
- developing assisted living facilities in collaboration with experienced developers and operators; and
- expanding and integrating home care services into the continuum.

STRATEGIC PLAN
IMPLEMENTATION

Acute rehabilitation and a skilled nursing facility were identified as priorities for SHS, and the case for action was so compelling that implementation was initiated even before the strategic plan was finalized. Because of the need to own at least some skilled beds, SHS purchased a nursing home in order to obtain the license.

Based on market and internal analyses performed during the strategic planning process, SHS determined that the next acute rehabilitation and first skilled nursing units should have 30 beds each. Further, it was decided that both units should be located within an acute care hospital.

Facility modifications, staff training, and systems development for both units were accomplished within four months. Following the required filings and site visits, approval for both programs was obtained and the programs were initiated.

Within six months, the acute rehabilitation was full and had a waiting list, essentially all from internal patients. Awareness in the market was at the point in which the potential for external referrals had been established. The program was well-received by the SHS physicians and program staff, and because of thorough orientation, almost all referrals to the unit were clinically appropriate. The diagnoses represented by patients referred met Medicare certification requirements for a DRG-exempt, and thus, cost reimbursed rehabilitation unit. The skilled nursing facility opened six months after the rehabilitation unit. The skilled nursing facility was successful, but had the effect of slightly reducing the acute rehabilitation waiting list.

Following establishment of these units, SHS leadership turned their attention to integrating all post-acute programs, in order to achieve the full benefits of delivering a true continuum of care.

Notes

1. HCIA Inc., and Ernst & Young LLP. 1995. *The DRG Handbook.* Baltimore, MD: HCIA Inc. and Ernst & Young LLP.
2. Chi Systems, Inc., 1997. Population-Based Planning Model.
3. Ibid.
4. Zedlewski, S. et al. 1990. *The Needs of the Elderly in the 21st Century.* Washington, D.C.: The Urban Institute.
5. Lewin/ICF estimates.

Case Study:
Behavioral Health Services

Susan C. Sargent

BEHAVIORAL HEALTH, composed of mental health and chemical dependency treatment services, has historically been set apart from the balance of medical services. Going back to the "ships of fools," when the insane were sent out on ships to clear the prisons and sail over the edge of the earth, mental health services were provided by freestanding institutions. Mental health coverage was excluded from original health insurance plans on the premise that state-operated sanitariums would care for these patients. Over the last 20 years, carve-outs of behavioral health services within health insurance plans have been popular, as purchasers sought to control the cost of these services.

More recently, the extent of behavioral disease in the population has been verified, and its role in exacerbating medical or surgical problems has become better understood. As providers increasingly contract with insurers and employers under risk-bearing arrangements, with incentives to maximize the health of their enrolled populations, integrating behavioral health services into mainstream medicine has taken on new importance.

The following case study illustrates how one health system formulated strategies to address the increased market opportunities and expectations in behavioral health services.

CASE STUDY: XYZ HEALTH SYSTEM

XYZ Hospital, a large, tertiary hospital located in the heart of a midwestern city, initiated development of XYZ Health System by acquiring two suburban community hospitals in the late 1980s. The three hospitals had only nominal behavioral health offerings, but were attempting to develop a managed behavioral health organization (the Consortium) as an outgrowth of a wholly owned, successful employee assistance program (EAP) and a partnership with a local freestanding, well-respected psychiatric hospital. Spearheaded by a strong, charismatic director, the Consortium was able to assemble an outpatient network, develop referral arrangements for inpatient services that involved both the freestanding hospital and local acute care affiliates, launch a 24-hour access telephone line, develop utilization management criteria and procedures, integrate the product line with its EAP, and secure several contracts with local employers.

XYZ Health System, along with several other local hospitals, owned Heartfelt Health Plan, a managed care company that competed directly with another provider-sponsored health plan in town, Moon Health Plan. Although Heartfelt Health Plan did not offer its own managed behavioral health product, its leadership had some concerns regarding the Consortium. Heartfelt worried that as the Consortium carved out part of the benefit plan, it could be a strong competitor should Heartfelt decide to enter this market. Further, the Consortium did not include all of Heartfelt's owner hospitals on its provider panel, which posed some political challenges for Heartfelt.

In 1992, stimulated by the entry of national managed behavioral health companies into the local market, competition in the behavioral health market intensified. Moon Health Plan and its owner hospitals affiliated with the local Blue Cross Plan, creating Blue Moon Health Plan, which decided to develop its own managed behavioral healthcare product. Blue Moon recruited the director of the Consortium along with the freestanding psychiatric hospital to join its ranks. XYZ Health System had never had a strong commitment to behavioral health and was now at a competitive disadvantage in attempting to compete with the hospitals in Blue Moon Health Plan, as well as proprietary hospitals entering the market.

XYZ decided to use Heartfelt Health Plan as a vehicle to strengthen its managed behavioral health products and also acquired a freestanding subspecialty psychiatric hospital that had a strong, regional reputation for treating children and adolescents. In addition, XYZ Health System entered into discussions with seven other hospitals in the metropolitan area to create a larger health system that could more effectively compete with the owner hospitals of Blue Moon Health Plan.

These discussions faced many roadblocks, including overtures from other systems for some of the hospitals and substantial conflicts resulting from differing religious affiliations. As an interim effort, the participants decided to undertake several focused studies in home health, occupational health, and behavioral health to identify the specific opportunities and potential vehicles for cooperation. These services were selected because the group believed existing programs could be easily integrated, and none of the services would require major capital investments.

Behavioral Health
Strategic Plan: 1994

Of the eight participants in the system discussions, only three had significant behavioral health offerings:

- XYZ Health System had a suburban inpatient unit, the freestanding subspecialty psychiatric hospital, outpatient clinics, and an EAP;
- ABC Medical Center had inpatient adult, adolescent, and chemical dependency units; several partial hospitalization programs; outpatient clinics; and an EAP; and
- MNO Medical Center had inpatient adult and adolescent units, several partial hospitalization programs, and outpatient clinics.

A behavioral health committee, with representatives from each organization, supported by consultants and legal counsel, was charged with developing a business plan for an integrated behavioral health product line. A key assumption underlying the process was that in the absence of a unified corporate structure among the eight hospitals, the behavioral health product line would need to be structured as a separate joint venture entity.

Key findings from the analyses of both the participating systems and the marketplace included the following:

- While the systems had similar service offerings, their service areas had little overlap.
- The EAPs were complementary and, if merged into a single EAP, would offer an attractive array of products.
- The systems had effectively downsized, cross-trained their staffs, and implemented managed care practices resulting in good inpatient utilization and efficiencies.
- Service gaps included medical-psychiatric capacity, geropsychiatric partial hospitalization, and adolescent chemical dependency programs, and the three systems offered a variety of unprofitable and redundant outpatient services.

- There was a significant oversupply of acute psychiatric beds in the metropolitan area, with half of them in freestanding, for-profit psychiatric hospitals that had recently experienced sharp declines in utilization.

- Four market trends were identified that could impact product line design: the growth of two competing integrated behavioral health delivery systems, the emergence of managed Medicaid gatekeepers, the growth of Heartfelt Health Plan and its line of insurance products, and an increase in risk-based contracting.

As part of the process, goals for product line development were formulated based on input from the participating hospitals, the behavioral health disciplines (e.g., psychiatry, social work, psychology, addictions counseling), affiliated organizations (e.g., Heartfelt), and employee assistance personnel. The committee agreed upon the following goals:

- maintain or enhance the quality of services provided by participating systems;

- operate within a corporate structure with the flexibility to provide a full continuum of services, assume risk, and allow for growth in ownership;

- enable the participating systems to reduce costs;

- ensure geographic coverage;

- maintain a strong relationship with Heartfelt Health Plan;

- diversify the revenue base by contracting with noncompeting organizations;

- facilitate integration of behavioral health services into the full medical continuum of care; and

- generate a return on investment.

A for-profit shareholder corporation was recommended that would operate multiple outpatient behavioral health centers throughout the metropolitan area and would be owned, initially, by three of the eight participating systems. Services to be provided by this new entity (New Behavioral Company [NBC]) would include contracting, planning and marketing, EAP, 24-hour crisis line, quality assurance and utilization management, data collection and analysis, billings and collections, product development, provider relations, and management of outpatient services to be provided at the centers. These services would enable the three-hospital joint venture to effectively compete with Blue Moon's managed behavioral health offering and position XYZ Health System to augment Heartfelt's overall medical plans with a specialty carve-out.

The strategic plan was accepted by the three participating systems and presented to the overall steering committee for incorporation into plans for the larger system. However, the eight-hospital system discussions eventually dissolved, leaving the three behavioral health participants back in the roles of competitors and putting NBC on the shelf.

Two years later, XYZ Health System and ABC Medical Center developed a joint operating agreement, forming Mid-America Health System. Behavioral health was one of the first initiatives undertaken by Mid-America.

Behavioral Health
Strategic Plan: 1996

The behavioral health marketplace had changed dramatically in two years. In addition, the entities originally interested in developing a behavioral health product line had consolidated, creating the potential for a wholly owned continuum of services and products. While the behavioral health goals remained much the same, changes to the marketplace included the following:

- Managed care development had proceeded primarily along PPO lines, as opposed to HMO lines. Restrictions on inpatient psychiatric admissions were growing more stringent with an increasing proportion of patients admitted with medical comorbidities.

- Relying on Heartfelt's sales, Mid-America Health System found itself participating on panels for only 45 percent of the population, whereas the Blue Moon providers had access to 63 percent of the population.

- The state mental health department had initiated discussions with acute care systems to privatize the care of its public mental health patients.

- Employers were beginning to consider direct contracting for selected specialties, including behavioral health.

- Population increases and aging of the population would increase demand for behavioral services, especially for patients likely to have comorbid medical conditions.

- While continuing to be overbedded, the freestanding psychiatric hospitals were approaching the acute care systems regarding joint ventures or acquisition. Community mental health centers were also exploring affiliation opportunities.

- Mid-America had developed a percentage-of-premium contract, which included behavioral health services, with Heartfelt for its Medicare population.

- Four managed care plans, with an estimated 250,000 covered lives, did not yet contract exclusively with either of the area's major provider systems.

- Heartfelt had been designated as one of four HMOs to serve Medicaid eligibles. Medicaid HMO contracts included behavioral health services. The Medicaid population was receptive to HMO participation and enrollment was ahead of budgeted levels.

In sum, both the aging population and increasing presence of managed care indicated the need for behavioral health services to be provided in general acute care hospitals, where behavioral healthcare providers could be effectively integrated with medical providers. Further, provider systems would need to be capable of contracting at risk for general health or behavioral health services, because some purchasers wanted to carve out behavioral health benefits while others wanted to contract for comprehensive healthcare services.

Mid-America formed a behavioral health planning committee and charged the group with developing a plan to implement behavioral health as the first fully integrated product line in the system. The committee, in addition to developing a business plan, addressed external communication issues (e.g., how callers would access the entire behavioral system regardless of point of entry), internal communications issues (e.g., how staff members could be kept informed on all system activities), and corporate education issues (e.g., how the system's corporate leadership could be made aware of, and become advocates for, behavioral health). By addressing these issues, the committee developed the business plan and laid the groundwork for its acceptance and implementation.

The resulting business plan included the following components:

- targeted a 40 percent marketshare for the metropolitan area; determined the capacities of inpatient, residential, partial, and outpatient services by facility and location; and sized individual behavioral health services by service area;

- designed a phased approach to reconfiguring existing services to achieve the needed capacity, by location, in three years;

- developed strategies for expanding existing services and augmenting the continuum through partnerships or the addition of new services;

- formulated managed care marketing and contracting strategies to achieve the targeted marketshare;

- identified infrastructure enhancements (e.g., information systems, marketing, quality assurance, human resources) needed to support the targeted service growth and related managed care contracting activity.

The committee recommended creation of a freestanding corporation (NBC-2), to be owned by Mid-America, which could serve as both a carve-out and carve-in, risk-bearing contractor for behavioral health services. This structure would accommodate other owners as the system grew and the development of statewide or regional initiatives. It was further proposed that NBC-2 be allowed to pursue contracts with any of the four purchasers who were not affiliated with provider systems and which might choose not to contract with Heartfelt. This measure was proposed to provide Mid-America with access to patients in addition to Heartfelt's enrollees.

Looking to the Future

The plan's recommendations were accepted by the planning committee, although there are several key issues to be resolved during implementation. Mid-America chose to maintain separate cost centers at the four hospital sites. Because the sites have disparate financial systems, it is difficult to produce accurate and timely financial statements and thus to track financial performance. In addition, different methods to determine expense allocations and contractual allowances have to be accommodated, as do variances in salaries and benefits, and billing and collection systems.

Other challenges to implementing the plan include:

- developing a management structure to coordinate services delivered in both inpatient and outpatient settings for different, albeit related, clinical conditions (e.g., mental health and chemical dependency), and for various age groups (e.g., geropsychiatry, child and adolescent psychiatry);
- overcoming competition for budget allocations, service ownership, and so forth, to unify the sites and services into a single program; and
- recruiting senior behavioral health professionals to fill gaps in staff, promote team building, and create a unified program direction and vision.

Finally, both behavioral health and corporate leadership are learning to appreciate the dynamic nature of behavioral healthcare and the market for these services. They realize that to maintain Mid-America Health System as a competitive provider of behavioral health services, future refinement and perhaps reformulation of the strategic plan will be necessary.

CHAPTER 12

Strategic Planning Processes and Approaches for the 21st Century

HEALTHCARE DELIVERY SYSTEM SCENARIOS, 2000–2010 · · · · · · · · · · · ·

I N T H E preceding chapters, the topic of scenario-based planning was described and its applicability to the healthcare organization's strategic planning process was discussed. As we look to the future of healthcare delivery in the early part of the next century and assess how to plan for the changes that are coming, scenarios can be helpful in thinking creatively about the future environment. Scenarios can also assist in framing the processes and approaches that can be used in successful strategic planning for this uncertain future.

Two similar, but slightly different, forecasts prepared by a national futures planning firm and a noted healthcare futurist are summarized below. These forecasts collectively define the likely range of what the environment could be in the next decade and lead logically into consideration of how to address the potential challenges. Because the scenarios were developed in the early 1990s, some of the time periods addressed have passed; however, the events described in the scenarios may still play out, simply in later time frames.

Five Futures

Bezold (1992) presents five scenarios developed by the Institute for Alternative Futures as part of a national study examining how healthcare leadership practices may change to face the organization demands of the next century.[1] Bezold describes the scenarios as thematic images that simplify many complex issues. He also notes that the actual future is likely to be a combination of these and other scenarios.

Scenario 1: Continued growth/high tech

Economic growth, while irregular, is persistent. Most Americans are better off, although the percent who are poor remain at levels of the early nineties. National healthcare reform did not occur, and federal expenditures have not kept pace. Most states have followed Oregon's lead in setting priorities on what services are available through Medicare and Medicaid. Biomedical advances have made it possible to predict and manage health and illnesses over a lifetime for those who are insured. Multispecialty physician groups direct most care that has become more efficient and effective. Hospitals are smaller and fewer, with the national complement of hospital beds reduced to 550,000 by 2010. Healthcare expenditures grow to 17 percent of the gross national product (GNP) by 2001, but decline to 15 percent as efforts to reduce morbidity and fully cure patients offset expensive life extension technologies.

Scenario 2: Hard times/government leadership

Tough economic times take their toll on the healthcare system. A depression in 1998 and prolonged recessions slow innovations in healthcare. The affluence of physicians irritates consumers, and scandals emerge about benefits given to physicians for bringing patients to specific hospitals. A political coalition of employers, healthcare reform advocates, and poverty groups make reform a viable issue, ultimately leading to greater regulation of physician business practices, prices, and clinical discretion. Reform efforts create a national reimbursement system with the federal government setting prices as the single payor, but giving states discretion over the types of care eligible for payment. The system enables Americans to "buy-up" for better and more costly treatments, and 30 percent of the population elects to do so. Heroic measures to prolong life are dramatically reduced. Formerly uninsured patients are better off because of emphasis on service for all.

Scenario 3: Buyer's market

The economy is growing well and technology advances rapidly. A growing dissatisfaction with healthcare leads to a dramatic shift in health policy toward market-based performance. A powerful coalition of policymakers, employers, and consumer groups are convinced that modest changes will not work, and the responsibility for health and healthcare expenditures should return to the consumer. Health policy is changed to make all individuals who were not poor or near poor responsible for health expenditures of up to 8 to 10 percent of their income. Medicare and Medicaid are adjusted to ensure that all poor or near-poor Americans have basic healthcare. Regulation of healthcare providers increases as systems are put in place at the state level to certify the knowledge and competence of providers. Consumers, insurers, and managed care plans shun providers who perform poorly. With many buyers paid out of pocket and ready comparisons of providers available, a diverse and active market emerges. Consumers with good health and prudent buying are rewarded with rebates or not having to pay out of pocket. By 2010, healthcare's portion of the GNP is reduced to 10 percent as a result of better health, better and less expensive diagnostics and therapeutics, and acceptance of dying.

Scenario 4: A new civilization

The nineties are a period of greater social idealism that is reflected in the market and public policy. National healthcare reform occurs following the 1996 elections. More effective managed care is evident, with leading HMOs increasing their focus on prevention. Social HMOs begin to flourish as the optimal vehicle for improving individual and community health. An employer-based insurance program, established by national policy, and enhanced Medicare and Medicaid are developed. Private insurance and public programs include regulations that support effective managed care, prevention, and community focus. Government policies encourage the development of outcome measures for all providers and services. Physicians, nurses, and other clinical care providers are recertified based on outcomes. After 2000, healthcare expenditures decrease as a percent of GNP.

Scenario 5: Healing and healthcare

This scenario shares many of the characteristics of the New Civilization scenario, but with a focus on spirituality and healing the ills of the world. Overall the economy experiences continuing growth. In the mid-1990s, access to healthcare is guaranteed through mandated, employer-provided health insurance and expanded Medicare and Medicaid. The national health policy is much more coherent and integrated with other key areas of policy at local, state, and national levels. Government policies focus on outcomes measures to identify the most effective therapies, providers, and institutions, and allow direct comparison between conventional and alternative therapies. Local healthcare systems become more coherent and effective. National health policy establishes insurance mechanisms that favor health maintenance and allow expenditures to be made on personal and community prevention. Hospitals focus on curing the body and healing the person. Healthcare composes about 12 percent of the GNP.

Four Scenarios

Coile (1990) developed four scenarios or sketches of the future for healthcare.[2] While these scenarios are the most probable, in his estimation, Coile warns about the "wild cards," or remote but possible futures with low probability, but potentially high impact, that must also be considered.

Medical breakthroughs scenario

Sustained economic prosperity and significant medical advances in cardiac, cancer, and AIDS care are the driving forces behind this high-technology scenario. Health spending reaches 15 percent of the GNP by 2000. Physicians split into two groups: hospital-based specialists and community-based primary care physicians. By 2000, half of all specialists are affiliated with academic medical centers and teaching hospitals with research activities that enhance specialists' practices and referrals. Few primary care physicians admit directly to hospitals, leaving admissions to specialists. Science and technology flourish as government and private sector research and development spending increase 10 to 15 percent. Reimbursement is a mix of fee-for-service, case-based, and capitation. With the high-technology orientation of care, specialists outearn primary care practitioners by 30 to 50 percent. Hospitals fall into the categories of low-technology community hospitals and high-technology specialized facilities.

Managed care scenario

Managed care becomes the dominant form of healthcare, with 90 percent of the population enrolled in some form of managed care by the late 1990s. Healthcare inflation drops to below 10 percent per year. Physicians reluctantly support managed care. Office visits increase, but fees for diagnosis and surgery are cut. Science and technology gains are achieved, but not as extensively as with the Medical Breakthroughs scenario. Research and development spending is moderate. Payment levels and prices are set prospectively as reimbursement shifts to capitation. Healthcare expenditures exceed 12 percent of the GNP by 1993, but then slow down. Hospital closures continue at a rate of 75 to 100 per year, and then taper off.

Reregulation scenario

Reregulation sweeps the healthcare industry, with hospital rate review programs implemented in many states and certificate-of-need programs revived. States choose regulation over reducing services or restricting eligibility for Medicaid. Physicians are a target for

regulation with a national price schedule for medical services enacted. Physician incomes drop 15 to 25 percent and then level off.
Some specialists lose 40 to 50 percent of their revenue. Science and
technology advances are restricted. Healthcare spending reaches only
12 percent of the GNP by 2000. Hospitals cope with strict limitations
on capital expenditures.

National health system scenario

A Canadian-model, national health system is established in 1999
when managed care and reregulation failed to curb healthcare spending. Physicians are not federal employees, but the federal government
is the only payor. A single set of standard physician fees is enacted.
Physicians join together in groups to pool overhead and income.
Medical and technological innovation is curtailed with private research and development spending falling 50 percent. Several years
before the new system is enacted, healthcare spending surges. Hospitals are aligned along a three-layer system of federal facilities. About
15 to 20 percent of U.S. hospitals are designated regional facilities.
Another 50 percent are named community care facilities, while the
remaining small and rural hospitals are designated medical assistance
facilities.

HEALTHCARE DELIVERY
CHALLENGES, 2000–2010 ∙∙∙∙∙∙∙∙∙∙∙∙

These scenarios are extremely useful in helping to draw out some
of the major challenges facing healthcare organizations in the next
decade. These challenges include:

Cost control

As healthcare's share of the gross domestic product continues to rise,
the pressure to economize and potentially ration care will increase.

Aging population

The graying of America will lead to increasing needs for healthcare
services and a greater focus on geriatric services.

Technological advances

More sophisticated technology will allow better diagnosis and treatment while continuing to increase costs, unless these technologies
replace existing technologies or significant productivity gains accrue
from new technology.

Pharmaceutical advances

Also holding the promise of significantly improved disease management or prevention (i.e., genetic engineering), pharmaceutical

advances will lead to major increases in survival rates and, eventually, life expectancy.

Alternative medicine

The growth of alternatives to conventional medicine, such as chiropractic, acupuncture, homeopathic, and nutrition treatments, bears watching.

Information explosion

More information that is readily available will have both positive and negative consequences, including improving providers' ability to deliver and manage care, but also increasing capital needs to acquire and maintain the new hardware and software.

Consumerism

As consumers become more knowledgeable about their health and healthcare delivery, they will demand more and better information from healthcare providers, and more sophisticated management of their healthcare by providers.

These 7 major challenges could easily be expanded to a list of 17 or even 70. However, this brief list serves as a starting point for any healthcare organization planning for the next decade by defining some of the potential environmental challenges posed by any of the scenarios described in the beginning of this chapter.

HOW TO GET THERE FROM HERE: GUIDELINES FOR HEALTHCARE DELIVERY SYSTEM LEADERS

Whether organizations use the strategic planning process described in this book or an entirely different process, the following guidelines should increase the likelihood of successful strategic planning and future organization vitality in the new environment.

Be flexible

The scenarios of the future illustrate that the environment and the particular challenges healthcare organizations will face in the next decade could vary tremendously. In contrast to the "one forecast–one future" model that has characterized healthcare strategic planning in the past and present, we need to move to a more flexible model. Consideration of alternative scenarios is one good example of this and contingency planning (described in Chapter 5) is another. While strategic planning cannot be so open ended as to allow for any possibility, it must become far more responsive to rapid and unanticipated change. In so doing, it will allow organizations to cope with a more complex environment, and prevent many healthcare strategic plans from being outdated or useless within 12 to 24 months of their completion.

Increase rigor

Healthcare strategic planning is, at best, in its infancy, and as a discipline needs to become far more sophisticated in its approaches and processes if it is to consistently deliver value to healthcare organizations. Analytical methods need to improve considerably to adequately address the current and future environment. Previous chapters have addressed such topics as competitive analysis, forecasting models, and the links between strategic planning and financial planning. These and other areas suffer from a paucity of analytically rigorous approaches and processes, usually rendering these subcomponent outputs inadequate or misleading. Healthcare strategic plans need to greatly improve the rigor of these analyses, adopting approaches and processes used in other industries, and not hiding behind inadequate data as an excuse for failure to execute this aspect of strategic planning properly.

Assimilate information effectively

Lack of data, flawed data, too much irrelevant data, and failure to use information technology effectively characterize healthcare strategic planning today, and handicap planners' abilities to be analytically rigorous and apply appropriate process techniques. Data problems can be an excuse for avoiding new and complex analytical techniques. Healthcare system leaders must demand more from their staffs, and improve information and information processing, while at the same time improve the analytical and process approaches to which they relate.

Improve process

Much of this book is devoted to process approaches and techniques to use in healthcare strategic planning because successful healthcare strategic planning is overwhelmingly dependent on good process. And, with the growing complexity of the healthcare environment and challenges, the importance of a solid planning process is unlikely to diminish in the foreseeable future. Good process enables the organization to move forward and manage the changes it creates and encounters effectively. One of the principal opportunities for healthcare strategic planning in the next decade is to increase the application of proven, more sophisticated process approaches used in other industries, including those involving information technology.

APPROACHING THE 21ST CENTURY

The good old days of the relatively calm and stable healthcare environment are long gone. Intuition and educated guesses are no longer viable substitutes for sound planning methods. Change is occurring so rapidly that it is impossible to fully understand its scope and impact. With organizations no longer able to rely on the accuracy of long-range forecasts, they must improve their ability to respond to unanticipated changes in the market.

The question is, how will change be experienced. According to Hamel and Prahalad (1994), organizations have two choices: "Given that change is inevitable, the real issue for managers is whether that change will happen belatedly, in a crisis atmosphere, or with foresight, in a calm and considered manner; whether the transformation agenda will be set by a company's more prescient competitors or by its own point of view; whether the transformation will be spasmodic and brutal or continuous and peaceful."[3]

To quote George Bernard Shaw, "To be in hell is to drift, to be in heaven is to steer." Strategic planning is the vehicle that enables healthcare organizations to steer and have control over their futures. Yet, strategic planning is a journey without a specific destination. It will take soul-searching, courage, and commitment to face a future full of uncertainty and potential threats. Strategic planning can be the road map to guide organizations through the unknown, balancing the need for articulated and compelling vision and direction with the flexibility to adapt and respond as healthcare is transformed for the twenty-first century.

Notes

1. Bezold, C. 1992. "Five Futures." *Healthcare Forum.* 35 (3): 29–42.
2. Coile, R. 1990. *The New Medicine: Reshaping Medical Practice and Health Care Management.* Rockville, MD: Aspen Publishers, Inc.
3. Hamel, G., and C. K. Prahalad. 1994. "Competing for the Future." *Harvard Business Review.* 72 (4): 128.

About the Authors

Alan M. Zuckerman, FAAHC, CHE, is a founding partner and director of Health Strategies & Solutions, Inc., a leading national healthcare consulting firm. Mr. Zuckerman has been a management consultant for 25 years, working exclusively for healthcare providers across the United States.

During his career, Mr. Zuckerman's consulting work has focused on strategic planning with this book being an outgrowth of his experience with hundreds of diverse healthcare organizations. Among his strategic planning clients have been large and small community hospitals, academic medical centers, single and multispecialty physician groups, nursing homes, retirement centers, hospices, home care agencies, and psychiatric and rehabilitation specialty centers. In recent years, he has concentrated on assisting clients with development of integrated delivery systems.

Mr. Zuckerman is widely published and a frequent speaker at national healthcare conferences. He is a fellow of the American Association of Healthcare Consultants, a diplomate of the American College of Healthcare Executives, and a member of the Society for Healthcare Strategy and Market Development and the Society for Ambulatory Care Professionals.

Mr. Zuckerman is married with two children. He is a native of New York and has resided in Philadelphia for the past 25 years.

Susan C. Sargent, CMC, is president of Sargent & Associates, a management consulting firm specializing in healthcare strategic planning, behavioral health, and clinical service line integration. She was previously a vice president at Chi Systems, Inc., and served as the firm's national director of behavioral health consulting services. Prior to joining Chi Systems, she was founder and president of GLS Associates, Inc. Ms. Sargent has over 20 years of experience in behavioral healthcare consulting, emphasizing strategic planning, management and financing of mental health and substance abuse services, managed care planning, development of alternative delivery systems, and negotiation of managed care contracts. She has a master's degree in business administration from the Wharton School of the University of Pennsylvania and a bachelor of arts degree from Smith College.

Karl G. Bartscht, FAAHC, CHE, is chairman of the Chi Systems Division of Superior Consultant Company, Inc., a healthcare consulting firm. Mr. Bartscht is nationally recognized as a pioneer in healthcare consulting and management, with over 30 years of experience in the healthcare field. He has assisted a variety of clients in developing programs and services that enable diversification into various post-acute markets. Mr. Bartscht also has considerable experience in direct administration of post-acute services. He has been involved in the development and management of subacute care and rehabilitation units as well as program planning and implementation services for such facilities.

Justin E. Doheny, CHE, is executive vice president and chief operating officer of St. Peter's Medical Center in New Brunswick, New Jersey. For the preceding ten years, he served as president of Wayne General Hospital in Wayne, New Jersey.

Mr. Doheny has been a member of management teams at Monmouth Medical Center, Long Branch, New Jersey, the University of Nebraska Medical Center, Omaha, and University of Michigan Hospital in Ann Arbor. He held a variety of line and staff positions including responsibility for strategic planning, marketing, and facilities planning.

Mr. Doheny is a diplomate of the American College of Healthcare Executives. He holds a master's degree in healthcare administration from the University of Minnesota and a bachelor of arts degree from the College of Holy Cross.